Prevention

PART-TIME
Intermittent Fasting

ABOUT THE AUTHORS

BRIERLEY HORTON, M.S., R.D.

As a content creator, Brierley Horton aims to inspire people to live their healthiest lives. And most days, she follows an intermittent fasting regime. She's a registered dietitian nutritionist with a master's degree from the Friedman School at Tufts University. She's also a mental health advocate and co-host of the *Happy Eating* podcast, which breaks down the connection between food, lifestyle, and mental wellness each week.

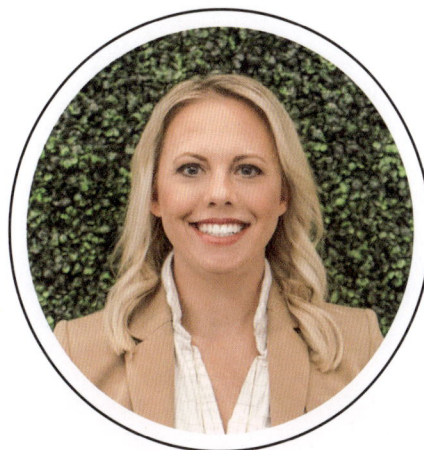

CAROLYN WILLIAMS, PH.D, R.D.

Carolyn Williams is a leading culinary nutrition expert and 2017 James Beard Journalism Award winner who's developed a knack for breaking down complex science into quick, reader-friendly tips. The author of two cookbooks, *Meals That Heal: 100+ Everyday Anti-Inflammatory Recipes in 30 Minutes or Less* (Tiller Press, June 2019) and *Meals that Heal—One Pot* (The Experiment, September 2022), Carolyn is a sought-after expert on anti-inflammatory eating and managing chronic inflammation through lifestyle. Carolyn writes on a variety of health and nutrition topics, and her work is regularly featured in print and online for lifestyle brands and media outlets such as *EatingWell*, *Real Simple*, *CookingLight*, and *Allrecipes*. She also co-hosts the *Happy Eating* podcast with Brierley Horton, M.S., R.D.

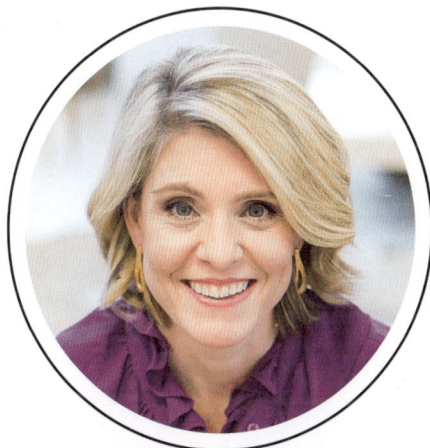

TABLE OF CONTENTS

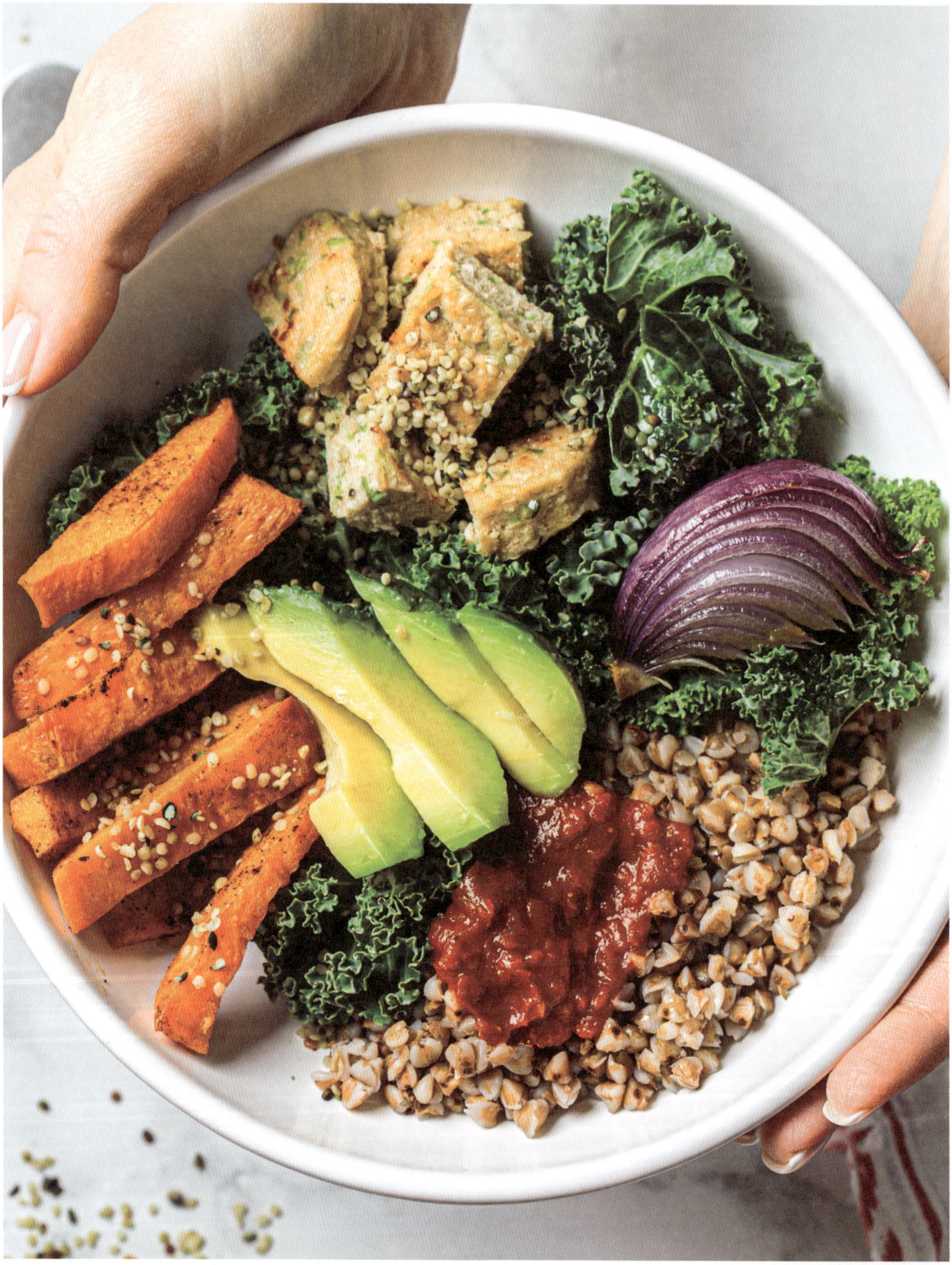

INTRODUCTION

I've always felt that eating is one of life's greatest pleasures.

There is so much delicious food in the world: I could eat an apple every day and not get bored. I've been handed down the world's best brownie recipe. I don't engage in the Chicago vs New York pizza debate because they are two different, equally mouthwatering foods. I cannot go to the farmers' market with just one reusable bag. In short: I want it all.

So when I first heard about the concept of intermittent fasting a few years ago, all I heard was fasting and all I thought was *nope*.

Then I learned more about it. It's part of my job to dig deeper into health trends, to ask questions and keep an open mind so that I can share the best possible advice with *Prevention* readers. So despite that initial reaction, I did that.

As I talked to experts (nutritionists, doctors, longevity researchers, brain health scientists, and more), I was impressed. There are a lot of benefits to intermittent fasting that you'll read about in this book—and yes, weight loss is one of them. But I also discovered, to my great delight, that there's a way to do intermittent fasting that doesn't truly feel like *fasting*—so of course, that's what we're recommending in this book.

When you do intermittent fasting our way, I think you'll find that you become more mindful of what you eat, and that may be the most powerful effect of all. As I've gotten older, I've learned I can't just eat all the pizza and brownies there are. There's the weight issue, for sure, but I also feel sluggish when I'm not mixing them with apples and farmers' market greens (and eggs! Oh, the fresh eggs!). When I put parameters around when I eat, it helps me think more clearly about what I want to eat: What

is going to keep me energized? What is going to make me feel good right now and all day? The answers to those questions change every day, but I'm always thinking about my food in a positive, productive way.

This book can help you do that, and give you the tools and recipes to enjoy every single bite, every single day, while boosting your health and losing weight. Let's eat!

Sarah

Sarah Smith
Editor-in-Chief, *Prevention*

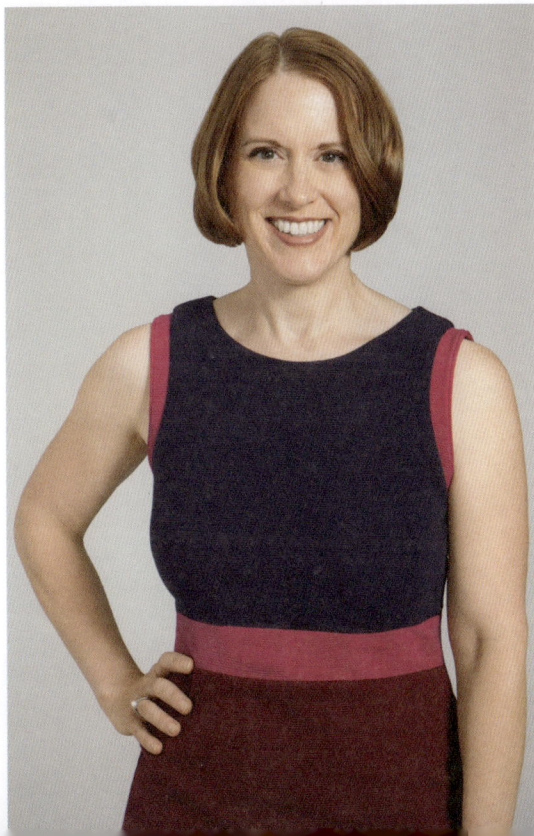

CHAPTER 1

Intermittent Fasting 101

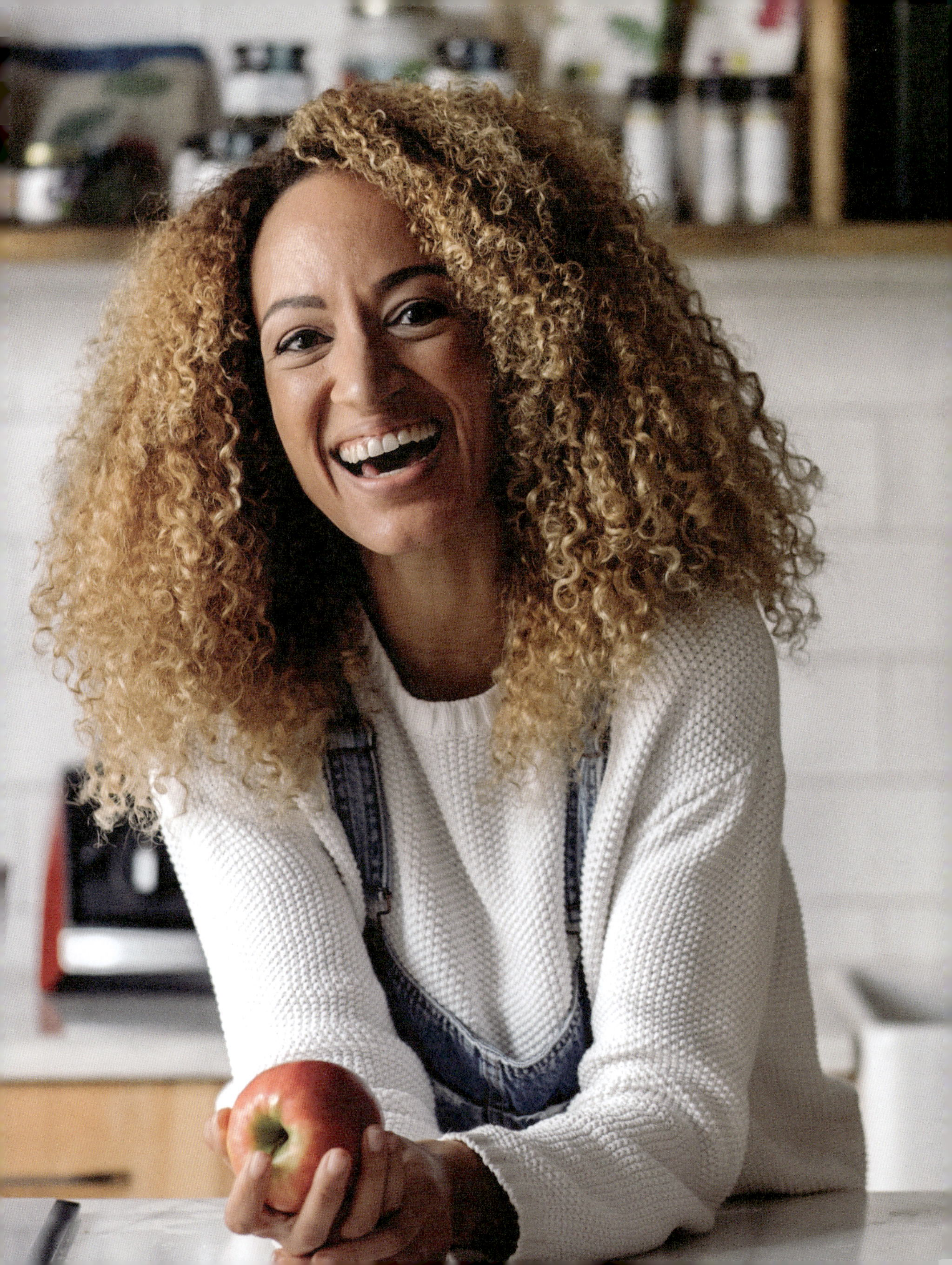

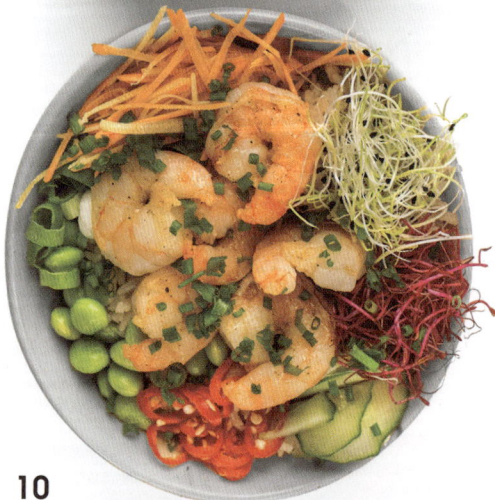

It may seem like fasting burst onto the wellness scene only recently, but the practice of fasting for religious or spiritual reasons actually dates back to prehistoric times.

Where exactly it originated is not fully known, but mentions of it are in many religious texts including the Bible and the Qu'ran. Today, fasting is a full-blown diet trend: The hashtag #intermittentfasting has over 100 million views on TikTok, according to one source. And in recent years, intermittent fasting has outpaced popular food trends like clean eating and keto. People who swear by intermittent fasting as an effective way to lose weight also say it has helped them feel healthier overall.

But What Is Intermittent Fasting?

There are different types of intermittent fasting, but they all adhere to the same overarching concept: Eat pretty much what you want, but only during a specific period of the day.

If you're the type to enjoy a bag of microwave popcorn while binge-watching episodes of the latest Netflix craze right before bed, the idea of ending your eating period much earlier in the day may come off as an impossible feat at first. But before you abandon the idea of fasting completely, we're here to show you how easy it is to start—and thrive in—your fasting journey, and still have the occasional late(ish)-night snack.

Intermittent fasting doesn't have a single standard definition or regimen. Instead, there are a handful of intermittent fasting methods, the most popular of which are listed below.

ALTERNATE-DAY FASTING This method calls for fasting from all food for 24 hours a few times a week, and up to every other day. Some people choose to eat a very limited number of calories on their fast days (usually 25% of your total daily calorie target) while others abstain from food and drink altogether.

TIME-RESTRICTED FASTING This type of fasting limits eating to within a certain window of time each day. It calls for fasting anywhere from 12 to 20 hours daily and eating within a 4- to 12-hour window. One of the most popular types of time-restricted fasting is the 16:8 diet (or 16:8 fasting)—it's where you limit your food intake to an eight-hour eating window and go 16 hours without eating any food.

5:2 FASTING The 5:2 method involves eating regularly for five days and fasting for two nonconsecutive days. On your two fasting days, you restrict calories to just 500 to 600. The advantage of following the 5:2 diet versus a time-restricted fasting plan like the 16:8 diet is that you can eat your regular diet on any day you want, depending on your schedule.

These methods, however, can be very restrictive, making it difficult for people just starting out in their intermittent fasting journey to stick to it. What we recommend instead is a method that may work better, particularly for women.

CRESCENDO FASTING This method calls for fasting for 12 to 16 hours at a time on two to three nonconsecutive days per week. And yes, a big chunk of that time includes bedtime. You can fast on a Monday-Wednesday-Friday or Tuesday-Thursday-Saturday schedule, for example. The meal plan in Chapter 4 is designed with a Tuesday-Thursday-Saturday fasting schedule.

Why Do We Love Crescendo Fasting?

Unlike other forms of fasting, crescendo fasting allows for shorter periods of fasting. And that's a good thing because "some studies have suggested that women may be more susceptible to the negative effects of prolonged fasting, such as disruptions to hormonal balance and changes in menstrual cycles," says Amanda Nighbert, R.D., intermittent fasting expert and creator of the Living Energized and Nourished (LEAN) Program.

Hormones play an important role in the way our body works. As part of our endocrine system, they're the chemical messengers in our blood that control many of our body's most important functions—from how fast our hair grows to our ability to lose weight. As we get older, even a slight disruption in our hormone levels can lead to more serious health problems.

According to a 2022 review study of human trials published in *Nutrients*, some methods of fasting may influence the levels of different reproductive hormones in some females, increasing estrogen in some, which is not ideal. "Women with higher circulating levels of estrogen have a higher risk of developing breast cancer," says Elizabeth Bertone-Johnson, Ph.D., an associate professor of epidemiology at the University of Massachusetts. This is a similar case for ovarian cancer.

Higher levels of estrogen also affect how our bodies deal with insulin, a hormone that manages blood sugar. Insulin allows the cells in our muscles, fat, and liver to absorb the glucose—or energy—circulating in our blood,

explains Cynthia Stuenkel, M.D., a clinical professor of medicine at the University of California, San Diego, and a spokesperson for the Endocrine Society's Hormone Health Network. When our estrogen levels climb, it puts a strain on our cells, and we can become insulin resistant, which means our bodies can't break down glucose the way it's supposed to. This turns into that stubborn belly fat that can be so hard to lose.

"Crescendo fasting may be more manageable for some women and less likely to cause these negative effects," says Nighbert. The advantage of this type of fasting is that it still restricts your calorie intake to help you lose weight, but because you're fasting for shorter, less frequent periods, it doesn't restrict calories enough to send your body into starvation mode and cause hormonal changes to happen. It's also a fasting method that's easier to adopt, stick to, and incorporate into your everyday life. And ultimately, that's the goal when it comes to weight loss and an overall healthier you!

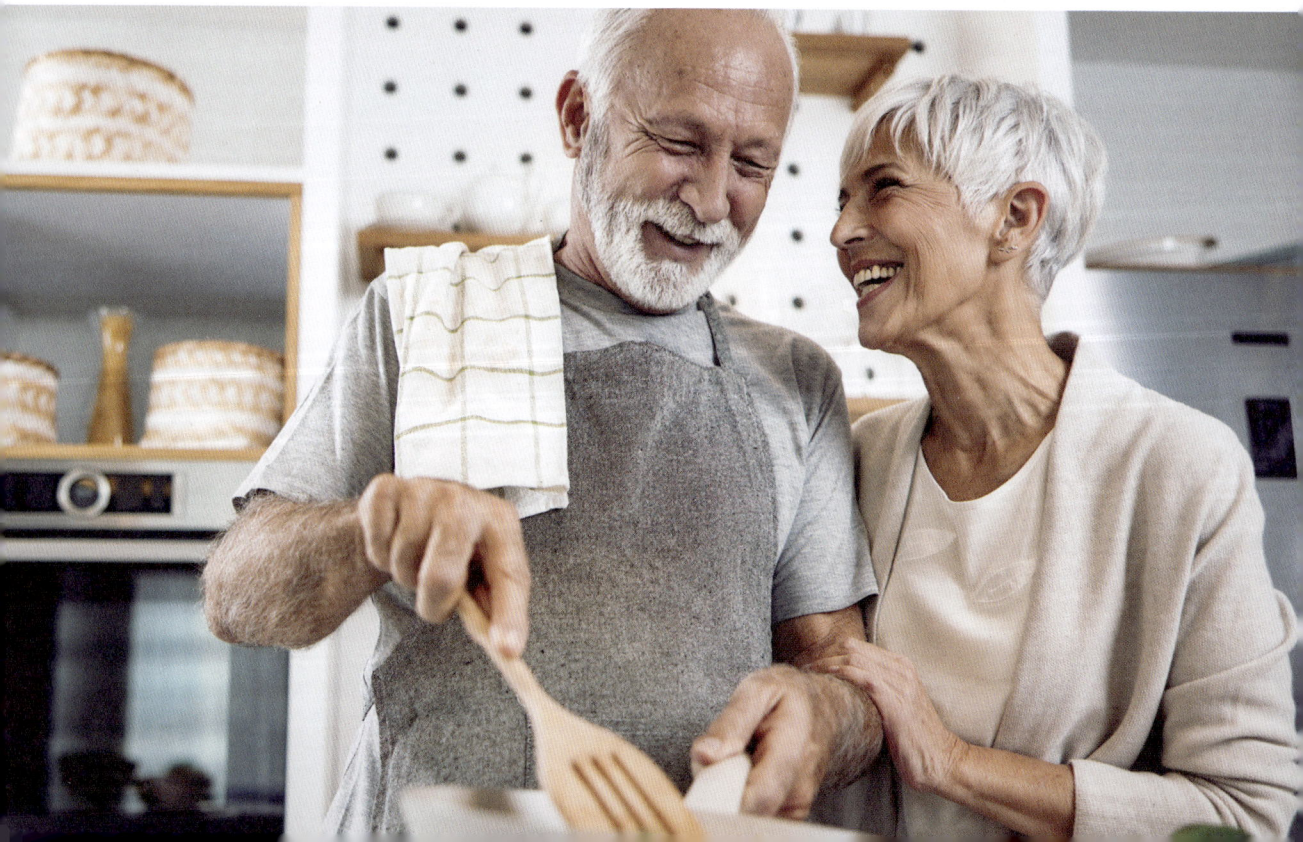

What Are The Benefits of Intermittent Fasting?

It's possible that part of why some people find the idea of intermittent fasting scary is that we forget sometimes that we already "fast" on a daily basis.

While sleeping the recommended eight hours per day, our bodies are not consuming calories, which is why we start the next day with breakfast: We are breaking our fast. Researchers believe the body truly goes into fasting mode—using body fat and ketones for energy—and cravings are likely reduced after about 12 hours. By ending our eating period just two hours prior to sleep and delaying breakfast for two hours after waking up, we can already reap some of the benefits of intermittent fasting. While studies about intermittent fasting have been limited, there is some promising emerging science around it. Intermittent fasting may help you:

LOSE WEIGHT A review of 27 trials found that participants lost from 0.8% to 13% of their baseline body weight with intermittent fasting, with most of the participants keeping the extra weight off. Also, 16 of those 27 trials measured body mass index (BMI), a simple number that estimates your body fat, according to experts at the National Heart, Lung, and Blood Institute. If your BMI is high, you might have an increased risk of heart disease, high blood pressure, type 2 diabetes, and certain cancers, so it's encouraging to note that in those 16 studies, advanced genomic nutritionist at Nutritional Genomics Institute Laura Kelly, C.N.S., L.D.N. says the participants' BMI decreased by 4.3%.

While intermittent fasting can help you lose weight, other weight-loss methods, such as calorie-cutting, are equally as effective, says a meta-analysis published in 2023. The reason why intermittent fasting is effective for weight loss is because shortening the window in which you eat every day usually decreases your total calorie intake for the day, which over time leads to weight loss without having to count calories. When 23 obese adults restricted their eating to 10 a.m. to 6 p.m. for 12 weeks, they ate around 350 fewer calories per day compared to the control group, according to a recent *Nutrition and Healthy Aging* study. This resulted in a few pounds shed and a drop in their systolic blood pressure.

Intermittent fasting also promotes satiety through the production of appetite-reducing hormones. A 2019 study from *Obesity* suggests that intermittent fasting can help decrease ghrelin levels—the hormone that fires up your "feed me" urges—in overweight adults.

BURN FAT, INCLUDING AROUND YOUR MIDSECTION If you go without food for six hours or more, your body starts burning fat for fuel. That may help explain why researchers at the University of Illinois have found that people who fast every other day lose 90% or more of their weight from fat stores on their thighs and hips. The fat loss is a good 15% greater than what people attain on traditional, diet-every-day plans.

Intermittent fasting could also help target the fat specifically around your midsection. A 2012 study also at the University of Illinois, found that after eight weeks of alternate-day fasting, participants lost three inches from their waists, regardless of whether they consumed a high-fat or low-fat diet on their non-fasting days.

LOWER INFLAMMATION Chronic inflammation is associated with a long list of health conditions, including dementia, diabetes, stroke, and heart disease, says Debra Cohen, D.C.N., R.D.N., associate professor in the department of clinical and preventive nutrition sciences at Rutgers School of Health Professions. While a handful of animal studies have shown that short periods of fasting (24 hours) lower inflammatory markers, the research in people is limited. Still, it's encouraging. For example, a small human study showed intermittent fasting reduced the levels of pro-inflammatory factors such as homocysteine and C-reactive protein, which contribute to the development of plaque in the arteries.

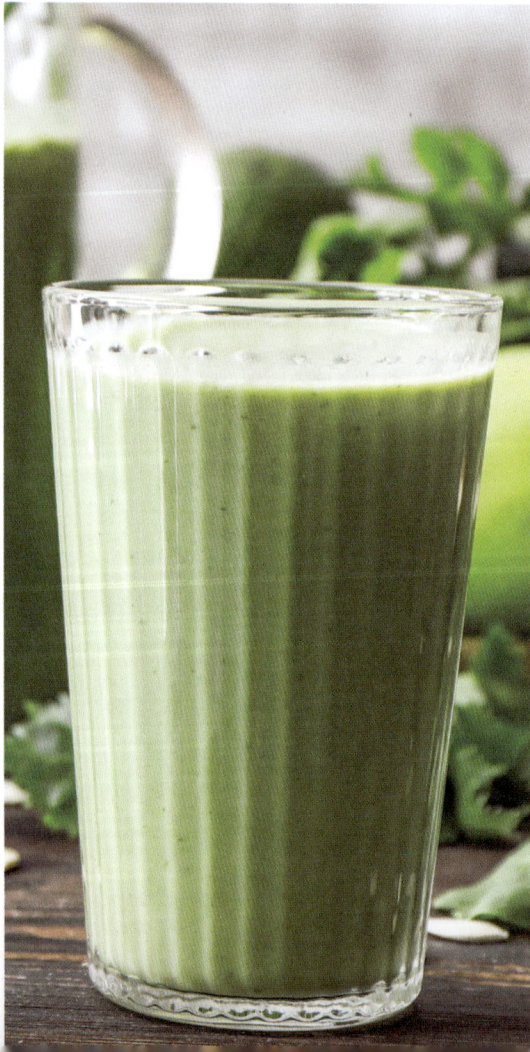

IMPROVE IMMUNITY Some research has shown that intermittent fasting induces a process called autophagy, which plays a role in the functions of your immune system, including cell survival, cell defense, and regulation of immune responses, says Kelly. For example, autophagy is necessary for T-cell production (a.k.a. the making of white blood cells), which helps your body fight off bacterial and viral infections.

LIVE LONGER Researchers are exploring how fasting may influence circadian rhythms to increase longevity, says Kelly. "If you think of all the molecular, cellular, and physiological processes in your body as functioning as an orchestra, then the master biological circadian clock serves as the conductor to make sure processes such as sleep, hormone secretion, metabolism, body temperature, and immune function occur at the correct time of day," says Randy J. Nelson, Ph.D., professor and chair of the department of neuroscience at the Ohio State University Wexner Medical Center. Circadian rhythms may become disrupted by age, illness, and environmental factors such as poor diet and stress. Studies have shown that fasting may optimize and "reset" these clock genes—thus helping you to live longer and also healthier. Put another way, your internal clock keeps ticking, adding years to life and life to years.

REDUCE CANCER RISK Intermittent fasting may also help lower your risk of cancer, particularly if you are overweight or obese. That's because fasting causes apoptosis, also known as programmed cell death. This means that your body is able to have more consistent cellular turnover, which makes it less likely for cancer cells to develop, explains Wendy Scinta, M.D., president of the Obesity Medicine Association and a member of *Prevention*'s Medical Review Board.

Moreover, a 2018 study from *BMC Cancer* suggests that short-term fasting may help breast

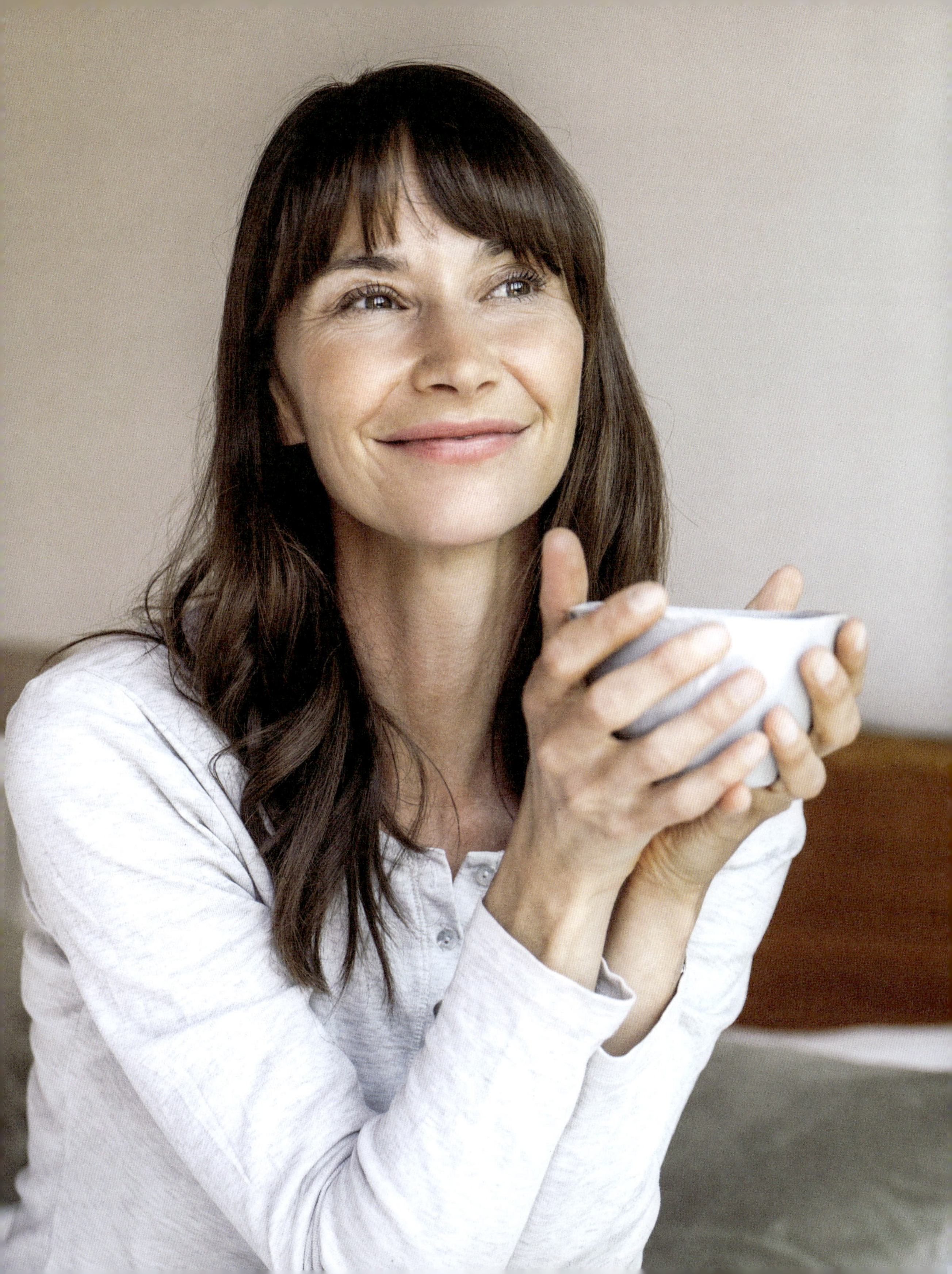

cancer and ovarian cancer patients undergoing chemotherapy tolerate treatment better and improve their quality of life. And because you'll have more consistent cellular repair, Dr. Scinta says you may have more energy too.

BOOST INSULIN SENSITIVITY Every time we eat, our body releases the hormone insulin to shuttle sugar from our bloodstream into our cells for energy. As we age, the body can become more insulin resistant, which means the cells in the body don't respond as they should to insulin. This messes with the body's ability to manage blood glucose, leaving blood sugar levels ever-so-slightly elevated around the clock, which is not only unhealthy, but raises the risk for future health problems such as type 1 and type 2 diabetes. If you're at risk of developing diabetes, intermittent fasting may help your cells become more sensitive to insulin, says

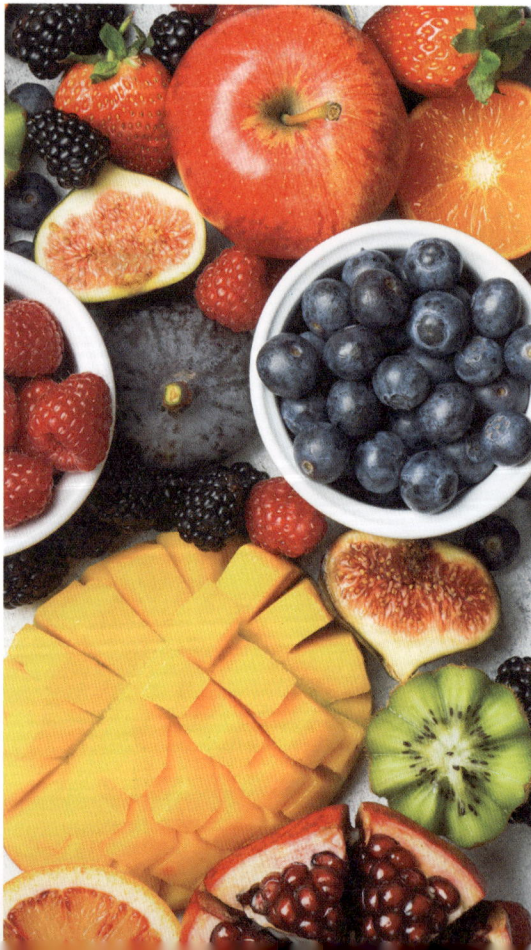

Robin Foroutan, M.S., R.D.N., a spokesperson for the Academy of Nutrition and Dietetics.

Insulin can also have secondary effects on other important hormones. In particular, leptin, the hormone that alerts your body when you're full, can be negatively impacted by insulin resistance. "Elevated insulin levels eventually lead to elevated leptin, as well," says Sara Gottfried, M.D., author of *The Hormone Cure* and *The Hormone Reset Diet*.

"Elevated leptin, despite what you may think, does not mean you are more likely to put down your fork and stop eating. Consistently elevated leptin levels can lead to a dysfunction of leptin receptors," Dr. Gottfried says. These receptors stop sending signals to the brain to tell you to stop eating. As a result, you do the exact opposite of what leptin is designed to control, and you continue to eat, never receiving the signal to stop. So increasing the time between meals can help because your body releases less insulin, which helps keep your leptin levels stable as well.

STRENGTHEN YOUR TEETH Every time you eat a meal, your teeth start the process of demineralizing, explains Mark Burhenne, D.D.S., founder of askthedentist.com. Demineralization is when your teeth lose calcium—it's the beginning of a cavity. "Whether you've eaten a carrot or a Goldfish cracker, the bacteria in your mouth excrete something that is low pH—or acid. This is called the acid attack after a meal," says Burhenne. After a little while, your body recovers, stabilizes the pH (saliva helps!), and your teeth start to remineralize.

If you are intermittent fasting, you're not constantly bombarding your teeth with food, naturally decreasing the frequency of demineralization and giving your teeth the opportunity to rest and stabilize for a longer period of time.

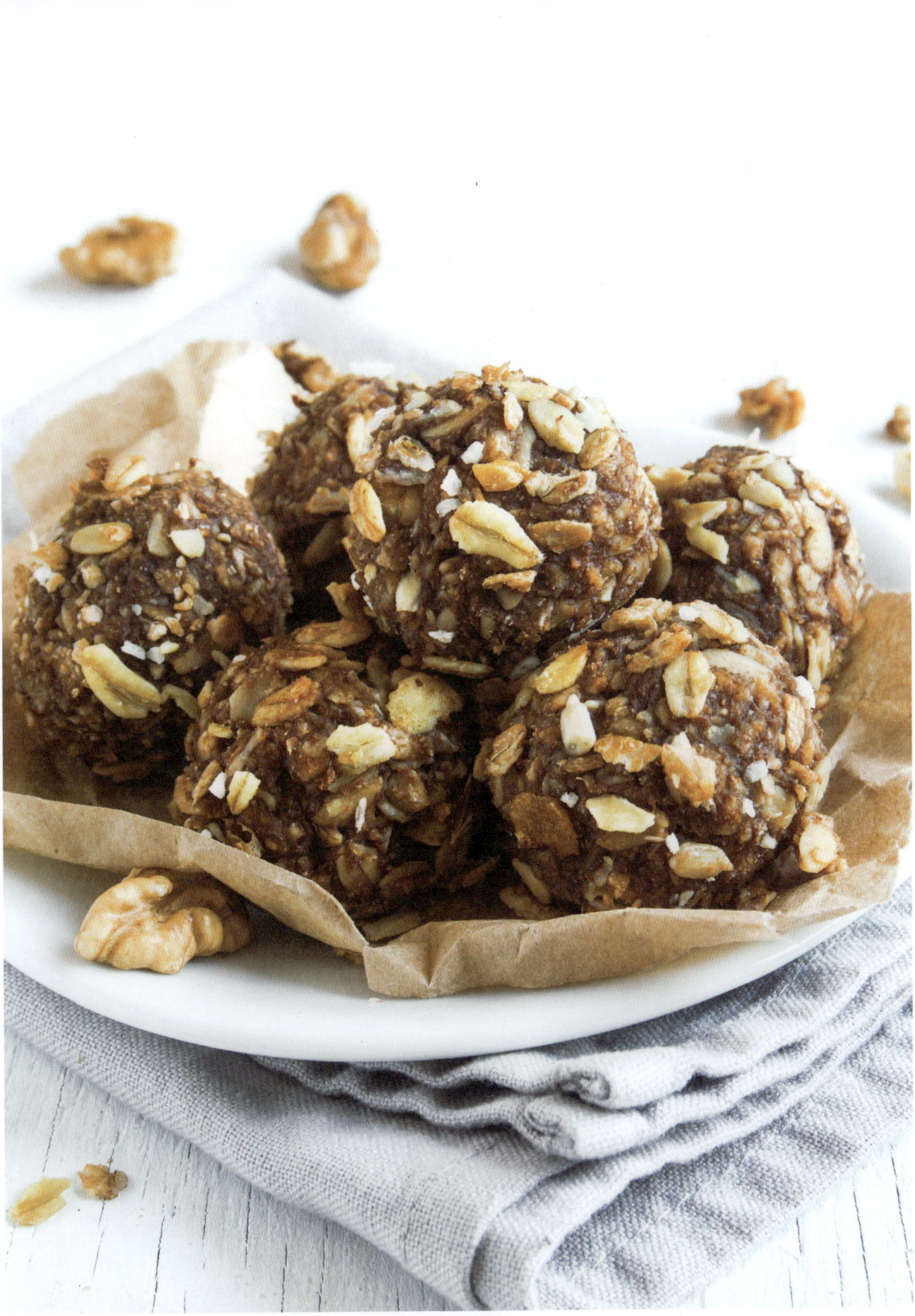

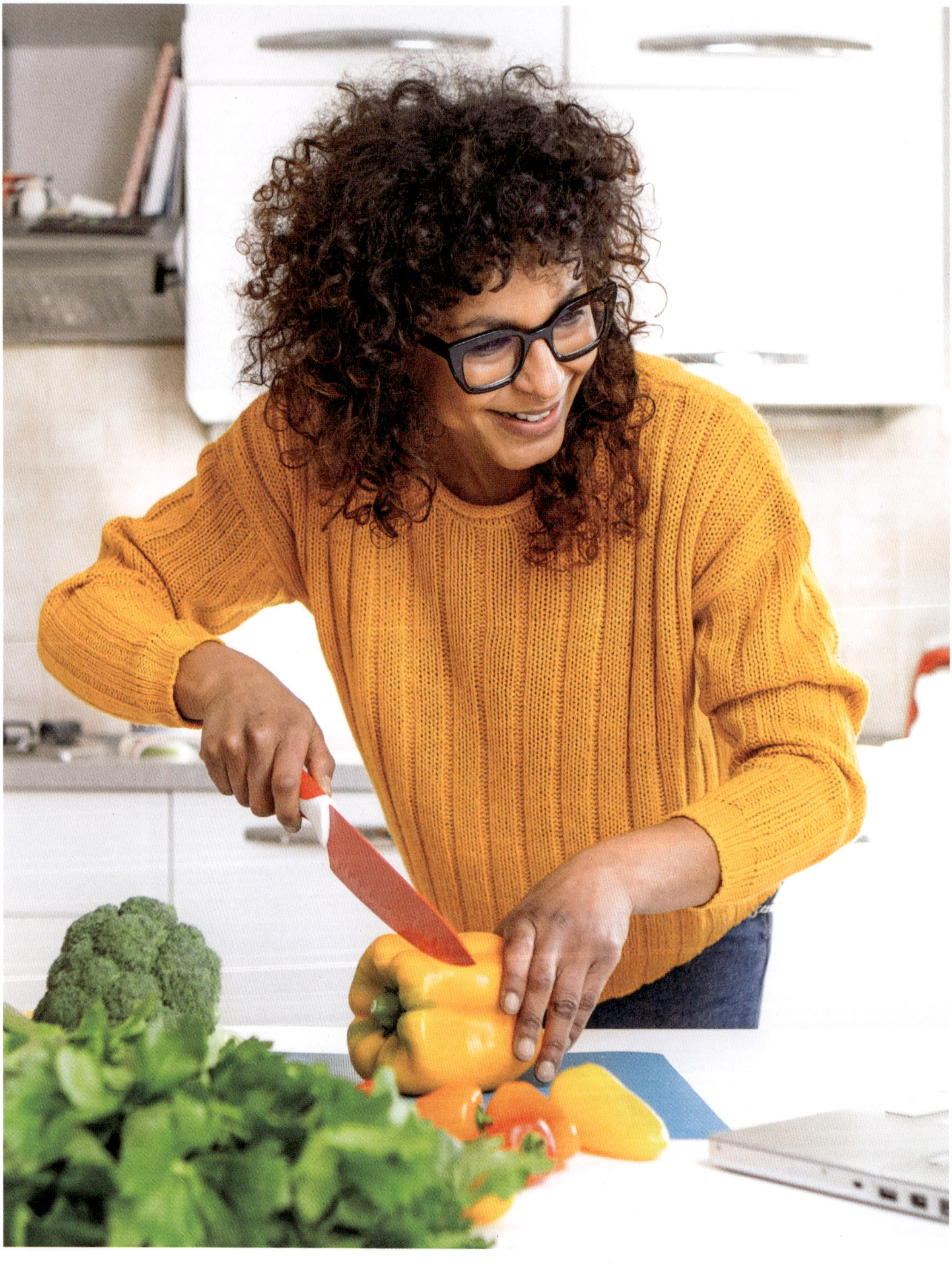

Who Should—and Shouldn't—Try Intermittent Fasting?

With a fairly extensive list of benefits to intermittent fasting, you may be wondering, "shouldn't we all be fasting, then?"

Unfortunately, intermittent fasting isn't for everyone. Some people should steer clear of intermittent fasting altogether. That includes:

KIDS AND ADOLESCENTS They require a steady supply of nutrients to support their growth and development—and intermittent fasting can lead to a reduced calorie intake.

PEOPLE WITH A HISTORY OF AN EATING DISORDER Fasting can be a slippery slope into disordered patterns, says Jessica Cording, R.D., author of *The Little Book of Game Changers*.

PREGNANT OR BREASTFEEDING PEOPLE Intermittent fasting can restrict intake of essential nutrients, which is not recommended during pregnancy or breastfeeding when a woman's nutrient needs are increased, says Nighbert.

PEOPLE WHO ARE UNDERWEIGHT OR MALNOURISHED The reduced calorie intake when fasting is not appropriate for individuals who are already underweight or are malnourished. For these individuals, getting to a healthy weight is important.

PEOPLE WITH CERTAIN MEDICAL CONDITIONS "Intermittent fasting may not be suitable for people with certain medical conditions, including diabetes, low blood sugar (hypoglycemia), or other metabolic disorders, as it can affect blood sugar levels," says Nighbert.

Taking medication that needs to be taken with food in the morning and/or before bed may prove to be tricky on this diet. Talk with your doctor or pharmacist to see if there's a way you can make your intermittent fasting schedule work with your medications. "Also, some medications, such as those for diabetes or blood pressure, may need to be adjusted if you're following an intermittent fasting diet," says Nighbert. Talk to your health care provider about how you can manage this while you're on intermittent fasting.

For most other healthy individuals who also have a healthy relationship with food, it's fine to follow a fasting regimen. "There's nothing really harmful in trying it if you have no underlying health issues," says Cohen. "And if it promotes weight loss, that can have great psychological benefits, which may spur you on to other healthy behaviors such as making regular exercise part of your life too."

People who are best suited to benefit from intermittent fasting includes those who are overweight and/or have high cholesterol (but are otherwise healthy), says Sonya Angelone, R.D., spokesperson for the Academy of Nutrition and Dietetics.

If you're ready—and cleared by your health care provider—to start your intermittent fasting journey, read on to learn about all the ways to make this transition manageable.

CHAPTER 2

Making Intermittent Fasting Work For You

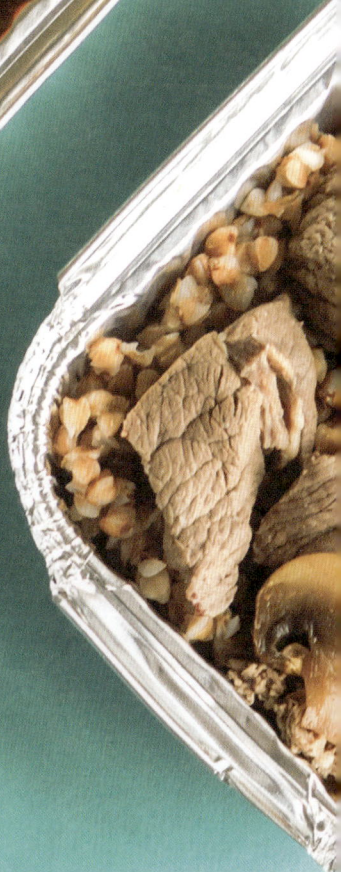

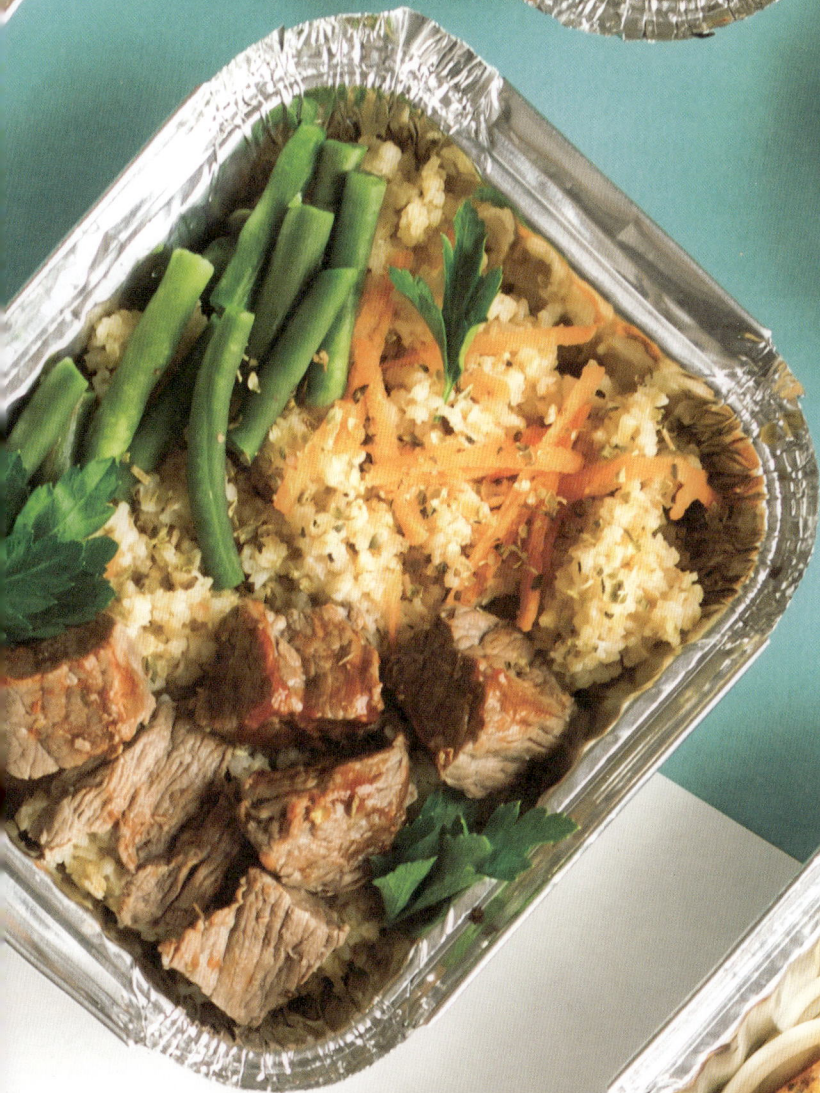

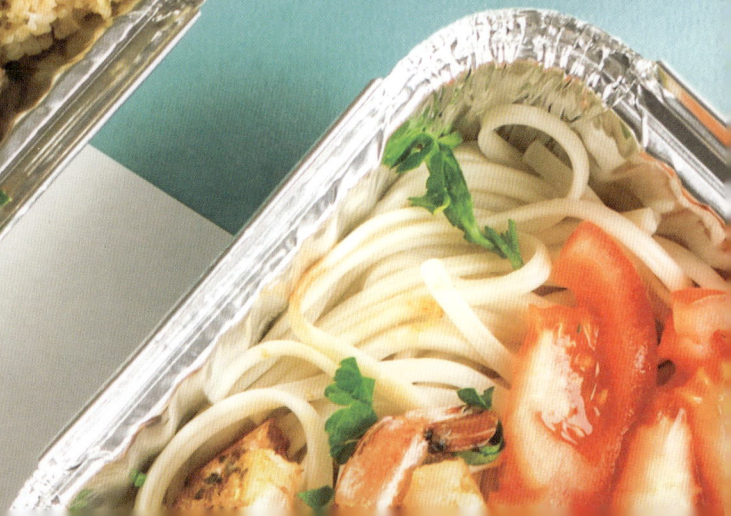

GETTING STARTED

Intermittent fasting requires discipline and a little background knowledge before jumping in with both feet.

One of the hardest parts of an intermittent fasting diet is getting started and training your body to eat within a smaller window of time. That said, there's no right or wrong way to begin your fasting journey. And starting on one day (like a Monday) versus another (like a weekend) won't make you more or less successful. We recommend choosing a start date where you can carve out a few flexible days in your schedule to make the transition to your fasting schedule. "If you're going to give this diet a try, cater it to your life," says Scott Keatley, R.D. of Keatley Medical Nutrition Therapy.

In this section, we share our best tips and tricks on how to transition to a fasting schedule successfully. But first, if you have a health condition or take a medication that may make intermittent fasting unsafe for you, be sure to check with your health care professional. "If you have conditions that affect blood sugars in general, you must make sure your medications are revised and followed. Also, those with unstable blood pressure should take into consideration the risk of dehydration and water fluctuation," advises Amy Lee, M.D., Chief Medical Officer of Lindora Clinic.

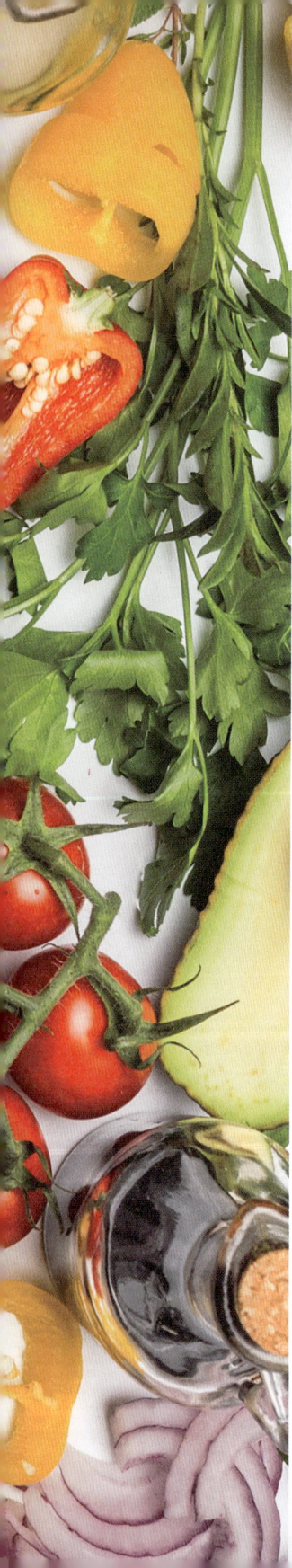

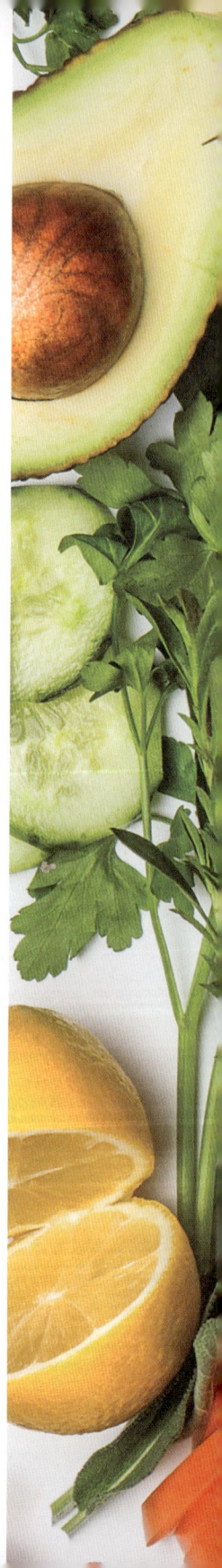

How To Transition to a Fasting Schedule—and Stick With It

To give you the best chance of success, we spoke with intermittent fasting veterans and here are a few tips they shared on making the switch and staying the course.

START SLOW If you plan to follow a time-restricted intermittent schedule—like the one we recommend—start first with a 12-hour fast and a 12-hour eating window. Then build up to a 16:8 schedule (where you fast for 16 hours and have an eight-hour eating window).

DEFINE YOUR PURPOSE Intermittent fasting can be a difficult eating plan to stick with if you don't have a reason in mind for following it. Keep that big why in mind at all times, and pull it out at the most challenging times. It'll help you refocus and push past hard times.

FEED YOUR MIND Read a book or listen to a podcast. Find mentally stimulating activities to keep you engaged enough to take your mind off your favorite binge-watching snack. You might also want to avoid any food-focused content. Simply looking at or thinking about food may make it harder to stick to your eating window; it might even trick your body into thinking it's hungry by releasing gastric acid into your stomach.

EAT BREAKFAST AS LATE AS YOU CAN Instead of breaking your fast as soon as you wake up, find activities to prioritize so you can push back your first meal of the day—do a morning meditation, take a shower, get ready for work, and then pack your lunch. Again, start slow, pushing breakfast back more and more each day.

EASE INTO YOUR FIRST MEAL Start with "something on the smaller side," says Cording, that also has a good amount of good-for-you fats, like nuts and seeds, that help prevent sudden spikes in blood sugar. For example, you can have a handful of almonds while you make a bigger meal to ease your stomach into eating again.

DRINK UP Your body can confuse being thirsty with feeling hungry. So when you're doing intermittent fasting, it's really helpful

↓

WHEN SHOULD I TAKE MY SUPPLEMENTS?

Take your supplements during your eating window (unless otherwise instructed by your doctor or dietitian). Most supplements like a multivitamin are better absorbed when taken with food. If you're taking a prescription medicine, talk to your doctor or pharmacist about the best time to take it with your new eating plan—some medicines are fine to take on an empty stomach (even encouraged) while others should always be taken with food.

to stay fully hydrated. Women should aim for about nine cups of fluid each day, but about 20% (or a little less than 2 cups) comes from the food you eat.

BE KIND TO YOURSELF "Intermittent fasting takes some trial and error—it's inevitable that your intermittent fasting schedule won't always go according to plan," says Charlotte Martin, M.S., R.D.N, C.P.T, owner of Shaped by Charlotte. If you're serious about continuing intermittent fasting, it's important to not feel guilty, ashamed, or mad at yourself when things don't go according to plan. Give yourself some grace and get back to a regularly scheduled program as soon as possible.

↓

SNACK WISELY

Smart snack combos that combine fiber-rich carbs with a little protein and fat help you sneak in needed nutrients, but will also keep you energized and satisfied until your next meal. Here are some ideas to get you started:

- Small banana and peanut butter
- Clementines and string cheese
- Almonds and piece of dark chocolate
- Toasted chickpeas or edamame
- Cheese and whole-grain crackers and grapes

Potential Pitfalls and How to Avoid Them

Just like any other diet, intermittent fasting comes with some side effects. Some are positive, like losing weight, while others can be challenging. Here we outline a few common pitfalls to watch out for and share tips to tackle or avoid them.

YOUR BLOOD SUGAR MAY DIP At first, you may experience lower blood sugar levels (called hypoglycemia), especially in the morning, which can lead to headaches, increased heart rate, dizziness, and nausea, according to Dr. Scinta. "When you don't eat, your body will first burn the glycogen (stored glucose) in your liver and muscles (hence feeling irritated at first), then it will begin to burn fat for fuel, says author of *Feed the Belly: The Pregnant Mom's Healthy Guide and Eating in Color* Frances Largeman-Roth, R.D.N. As your body adapts and learns to run on fat instead of glucose, hypoglycemia will become less common. This is a particular issue for those who have prediabetes, type 1 or 2 diabetes, or a known history of hypoglycemia, says Dr. Lee.

The solution: If you feel dizzy or lightheaded over the course of a few hours, Largeman-Roth says to break your fast and eat something—even if it's a small snack. During meals, make sure to fuel up on satisfying foods like lean proteins, whole grains, and healthy fats (avocados, nuts, and extra-virgin olive oil) to help keep your blood sugar levels steadier during your fast.

YOUR WORKOUTS MAY TAKE A HIT Following an intermittent fasting schedule and working out is totally safe, but you may need to make some adjustments to your workout routine

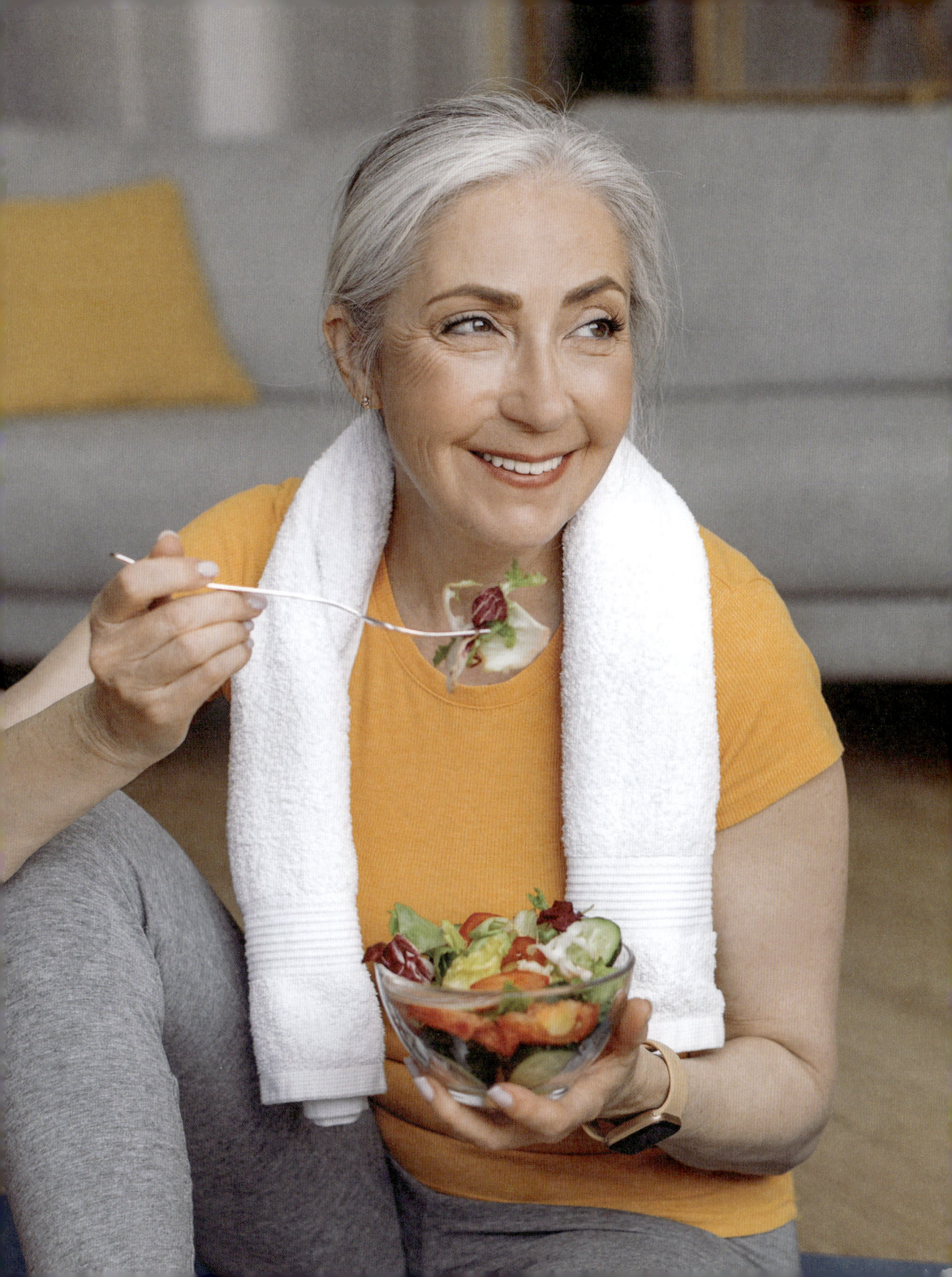

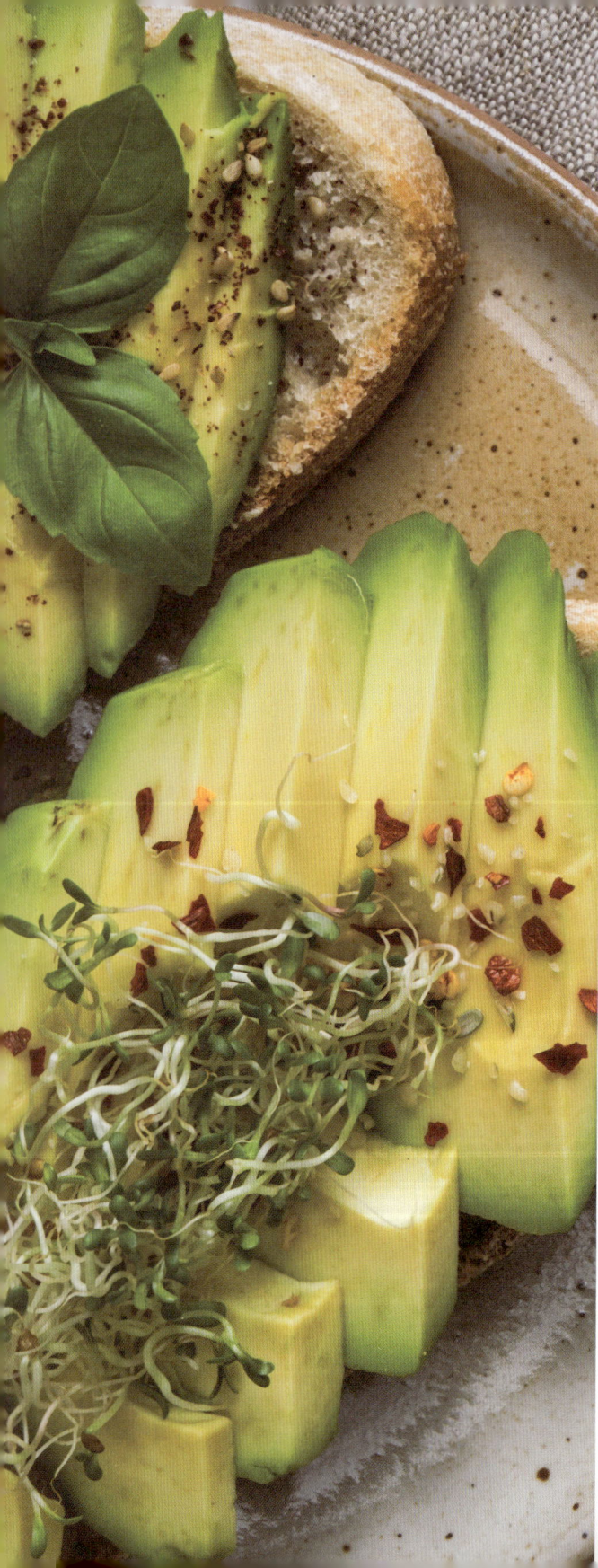

so that you still get the most out of it. On days when you're fasting, you may want to do a low-impact workout instead of a more intense one.

The solution: Dr. Scinta recommends timing your workouts so they're at the beginning or end of your fast. This way, you can enjoy a pre- or post-workout snack. Foods that are easy to digest, like a smoothie, low-fat yogurt, and peanut butter with toast work better pre-workout, while foods with a higher carb-to-protein ratio, such as a bowl of oatmeal, are ideal for post-workout.

YOU COULD GET OVERLY FOCUSED ON WEIGHT LOSS

Getting closer to your ideal healthy weight may feel great, but there is a tendency to feel like this isn't happening as quickly as you thought. So to fast-track losing those last few pounds, you may be inclined to eat less on non-fasting days. "When you don't consume an adequate amount of calories on non-fasting days, your body may conserve the energy you consume, rather than burning it," says Kristen Smith, M.S., R.D., spokesperson for the Academy of Nutrition and Dietetics. At the same time, skipping meals during your eating windows can cause you to be extremely hungry during fasting periods, making it more likely that you'll overeat when you break your fast.

The solution: Smith suggests making a meal plan for non-fasting days that includes balanced meals consisting of at least 300 to 500 calories per meal. In Chapter 4, we include a plan for your non-fasting days to ensure that you don't skimp out on much needed daily nutrients. You can also use this as inspiration for thriving in your fasting journey after these 28 days.

YOU MAY NOT PLAN HOW YOU'LL BREAK YOUR FAST

Planning out what you'll do when you eat again can help you avoid overeating when you break your fast. Also, since you only have so much time in your day to fit in healthy foods, it's best to focus on nutritious options.

The solution: Keatley recommends a complete protein that has healthy fats and is loaded with vitamins and minerals like eggs. "You'll also need to get about 25 to 35 grams of fiber [during your entire eating window], so including high fiber foods, such as beans, legumes, and anything ending in -berry is key too." Healthy oils like avocado and olive oil can also give you energy, he says. Then, Keatley recommends that you follow the same formula at your next meal, but with different foods.

YOU MIGHT FORGET HOW IMPORTANT SLEEP IS FOR YOUR SUCCESS Lack of sleep may disrupt appetite-regulating hormones, ultimately increasing hunger, according to a report from the American Heart Association. Ghrelin is a hormone that stimulates hunger and it increases when you're sleep-deprived. Leptin, the hormone that tells your body it's full and satisfied after a meal, decreases when you've been short on sleep.

The solution: Aim to sleep at least 7 hours per night to help keep hunger hormones in check.

↓

PRIORITIZE PROTEIN

People who are doing intermittent fasting often struggle to get enough protein, says Dr. Scinta, so remember to eat regularly, including snacks when you're not fasting. "You should aim to get at least one gram of protein per kilogram of weight daily," she says. A 150-pound woman is 68 kilograms (1 kilo = 2.2 pounds), which translates to 68 grams of protein per day. What does 68 grams of protein look like? That's 3 eggs (about 18 grams protein), a 6-ounce piece of salmon (about 43 grams protein), and 1½ ounces of roasted almonds (about 9 grams protein).

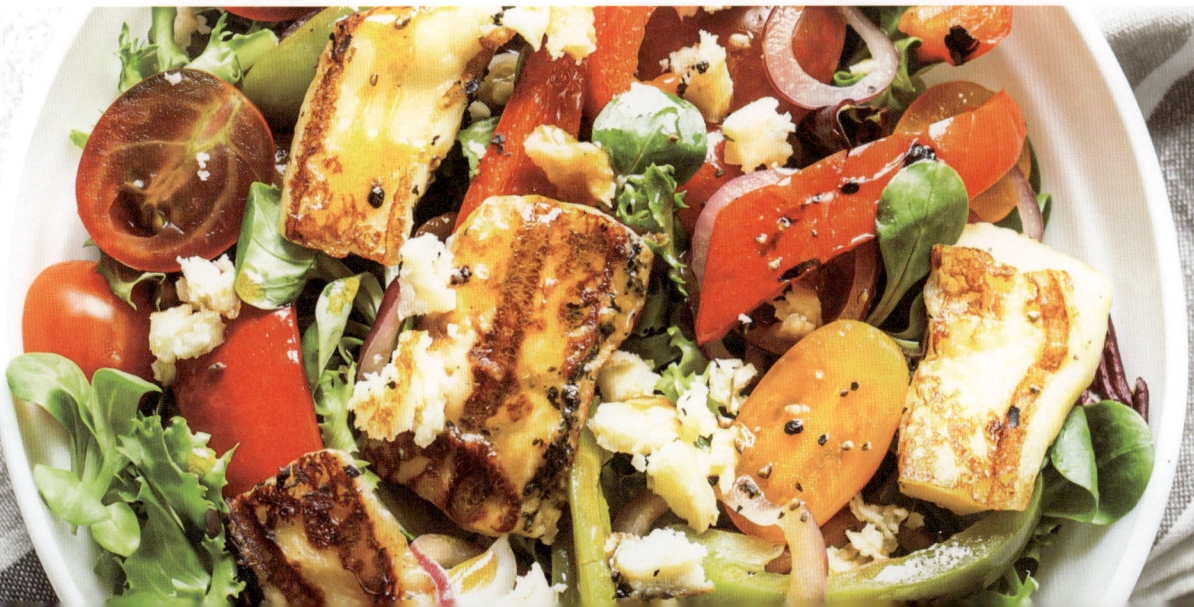

CHAPTER 3

How the Plan Works

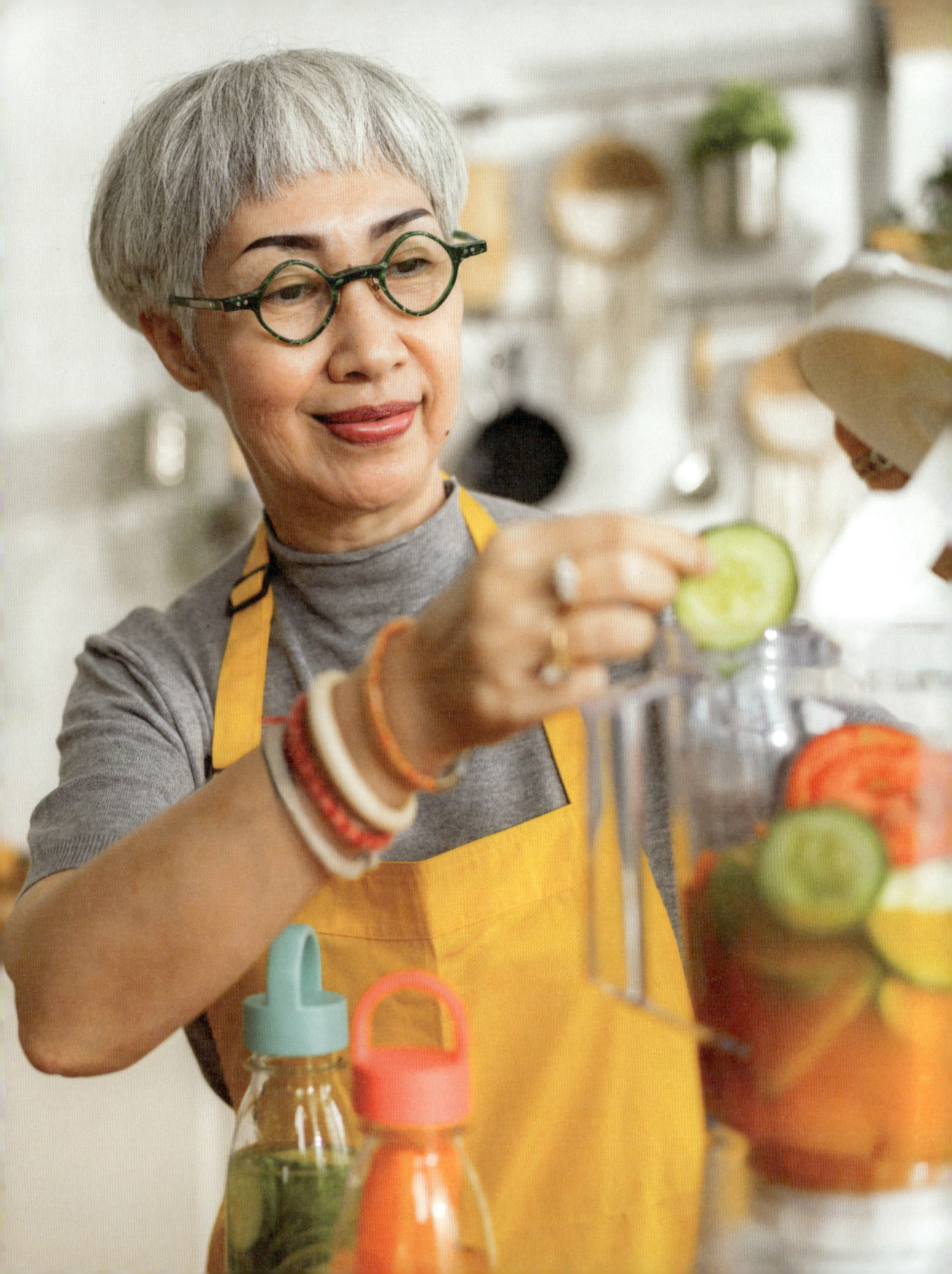

WELCOME TO YOUR CRESCENDO FASTING PLAN

As we explained in chapter 1, we believe this is the best way to start your fasting journey. Fasting for 12 to 16 hours on two to three nonconsecutive days per week is a more manageable method to adopt—and stick to—than fasting daily. You'll still reap the benefits of fasting without wreaking havoc on your hormones.

YOUR 28-DAY MEAL PLAN With a little bit of strategic planning, following our 28-day diet can be easy. The menus are designed around delicious, nutritionally balanced meals to keep you full longer, plus it includes healthy snacks for when you need a little boost. We've also included prepping tips to take the stress out of making your meals, as well as weekly shopping lists to make sure you have all the ingredients for a successful fasting journey.

Here's how it all works, so you can get started and stick with it:

HOW EACH WEEK WORKS You'll have four days with standard meals and snacks (breakfast, lunch, dinner, and two snacks). The other three days are designed to support a 12- to 16-hour (mostly overnight) fast that includes the same standard meals and snacks with the exception of breakfast. You will start your fast at night after consuming your last food or drink with calories, then fast through the night until late morning before breaking your fast with lunch.

For example, let's say you finish eating on day one at 8 p.m. Your goal is to fast for up to 16 hours, which would bring you to 12 p.m. on day two. Should you need to break your fast before then, you can move one of your snacks earlier in the day.

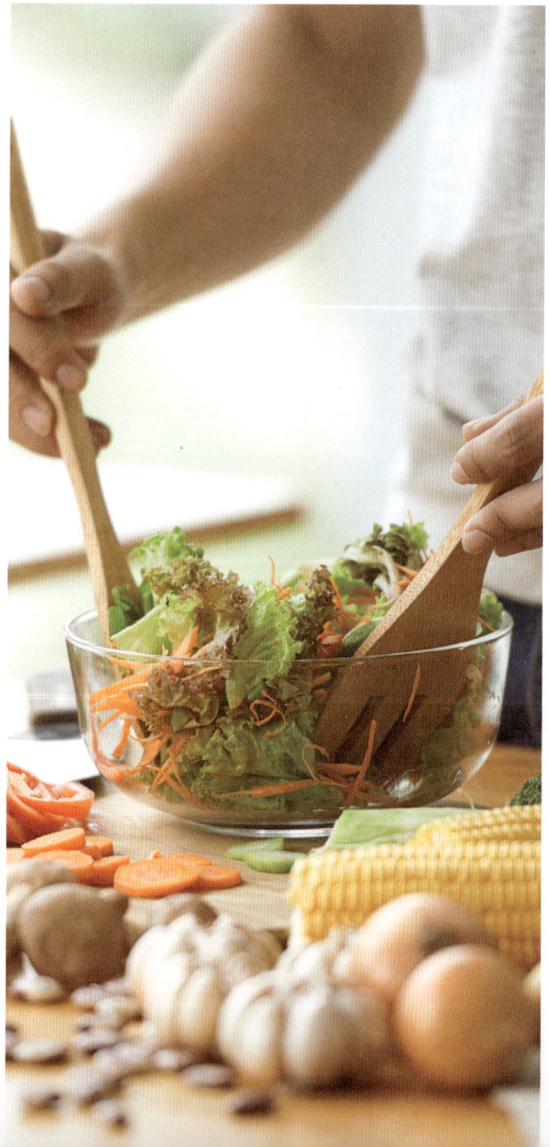

What your week could look like on this plan

DAY 1	DAY 2 (FASTING)	DAY 3	DAY 4 (FASTING)	DAY 5	DAY 6 (FASTING)	DAY 7
Breakfast (7 a.m.)		Breakfast (7 a.m.)		Breakfast (7 a.m.)		Breakfast (7 a.m.)
Snack (10 a.m.)	Lunch (11:30 a.m. for a 16-hr fast)	Snack (10 a.m.)	Snack (9:30 a.m. for a 14-hr fast)	Snack (10 a.m.)	Snack (9 a.m. for a 12-hr fast)	Snack (10:30 a.m.)
Lunch (1 p.m.)	Snack (2 p.m.)	Lunch (1 p.m.)	Lunch (12:30 p.m.)	Lunch (1:30 p.m.)	Lunch (12:30 p.m.)	Lunch (1 p.m.)
Snack (4 p.m.)	Snack (4:30 p.m.)	Snack (4 p.m.)	Snack (4 p.m.)	Snack (5 p.m.)	Snack (4 p.m.)	Snack (4:30 p.m.)
Dinner (last food intake at 7:30 p.m.)	Dinner (7:30 p.m.)	Dinner (last food intake at 7:30 p.m.)	Dinner (7:30 p.m.)	Dinner (last food intake at 7:30 p.m.)	Dinner (7:30 p.m.)	Dinner (8 p.m.)

HOW EACH DAY WORKS Each daily menu is built around nutrient-dense meals and foods to meet daily energy and nutrient needs. We took extra care to ensure this is the case on the three fasting days each week.

Daily menus range from 1,600 to 2,000 calories, contain a minimum of 60 g of protein, and do not exceed 2,300 mg sodium. On top of that, each day contains at least 5 servings of fruits and vegetables.

We built this menu to avoid drastic dips in calories so that regardless of when you want to throw in a workout, you're still getting adequate nutrition to sustain you for the day.

REMEMBER

Benefits to fasting are seen around the 12-hour mark, so you still have completed a successful fast even if you break it earlier than you intended. So, don't stress about it—it's normal to need a little time to gradually build your fasting "muscle."

FASTING FAQS

Can you eat whatever you want when you're not in a fasting period?

Intermittent fasting isn't a free pass to eat absolutely anything you want, contrary to what you may have heard (or wish were true!). You still should avoid processed foods and eat whole foods from plants and animals. Plus, you should aim to get moving for at least 150 minutes per week. "Your eating plan should be something you can follow for the rest of your life to promote good health," says Cohen.

What breaks a fast?

Some fasting experts will say you can have up to about 30 to 40 calories during your fasting window and it won't throw you out of a fasting state. Others say anything that delivers calories will break your fast. We tend to agree with the latter route and recommend staying calorie-free during your fasting window. That's because, as Cording points out, everyone's metabolism is different, so what kicks you out of your fasting window might not kick someone else out. "As soon as you consume enough calories to give your body energy to do anything, that brings you out of that fasting state because your body has been given fuel to work with," she adds.

Does the time of day that I schedule my eating window matter?

Some experts say it does. Keeping your eating window earlier seems to be the most beneficial.

The body's biological clock is primed to eat earlier in the day, explains Courtney Peterson, Ph.D., associate professor of nutrition at the University of Alabama, Birmingham. "In most people, blood sugar control is best in the morning and gets worse as the day progresses. You also digest food faster in the morning. So there's a metabolic advantage to eating earlier in the day."

Some experts suggest you begin your eating window at 7 a.m. and end it (a.k.a. start your fast) by 3 p.m. But for many that time frame is unrealistic, which is why we built our plan to begin a little later. And fortunately, there's science to support our approach: Other research suggests that bumping your eating window just a bit later, from 10 a.m. to 6 p.m., is also effective for weight loss.

REMEMBER
The best diet is one that you can stick with, and that means finding a plan that fits into your daily routine.

What can I consume during my fasting window?

Fasting by definition means you're not eating food, so this is really about what you can drink. You don't have to stick exclusively to water, though. Here are 6 drinks you can enjoy while fasting:

- Black coffee—hot or iced. Just skip add-ons like creamer, milk, or sugar.
- Unsweetened tea. Again, skip the creamer and milk.
- Herbal tea
- Sparkling water. Be sure to check the ingredients list to make sure there's no juice or added sugar.
- Zero-calorie drinks sweetened with stevia (also labeled as Reb A)
- Electrolyte water (smartwater or LIFEWTR)

Can I have alcohol on this plan?

It's generally OK to drink alcohol (in moderation, of course) during eating hours when you're intermittent fasting. That said, alcohol also has the potential to sabotage your efforts.

Drinking alcohol when you're trying to lose weight can sometimes hinder weight loss. The issue is mainly about metabolism. Your body sees alcohol as a toxin and prioritizes breaking down the alcohol. "The body has to sacrifice all metabolic process in order to metabolize alcohol," says Vanessa Rissetto, R.D., co-founder of Culina Health. This means your body metabolizes your food at a slower rate—and more of what you eat gets stored as fat.

And also, research has found that alcohol blocks fat breakdown, which counteracts one of the benefits of intermittent fasting—that it can increase your fat burn.

Can I combine this with other diets like keto or Paleo?

Yes, you can combine intermittent fasting with any other eating pattern that you like, including Mediterranean, DASH, low-carb, high-protein, diabetes-friendly, keto, or Paleo.

How do I handle fasting while socializing with friends and family?

The beauty of intermittent fasting, and crescendo fasting specifically, is that it's flexible to fit you and your schedule. If your social plans call for dinner, for example, line up your eating window that day to accommodate your reservation time. Alternatively, you could schedule social meals on days when you aren't fasting.

Is it safe to exercise while fasting?

Yes, it is absolutely safe to work out while doing intermittent fasting, even during your fasting window. You may need to make some adjustments to your schedule depending on how you feel. For example, some people prefer working out on an empty stomach so exercising toward the end of your fasting window would be ideal. Others have to have some sustenance in their system to exercise so timing your activity to be during your eating window is better. Maybe your timing revolves around the ability to have a pre- and/or post-working meal or snack. Pay attention to your energy levels on fasting days too. If you find your energy is lower on the days you're fasting, consider switching to a low-impact workout on those days.

Now, it's time to start your journey to a healthier you!

CHAPTER 4

The Meal Plan

STOCK YOUR PANTRY

Be sure to have these essentials on hand throughout the meal plan.

- Almonds
- Almond butter (or your preferred nut butter)
- Baking soda
- Balsamic vinegar
- Brown sugar
- Chia seeds
- Curry powder
- Dijon mustard
- Everything Bagel seasoning
- Garlic powder
- Ground cinnamon
- Ground cumin
- Ground nutmeg
- Honey
- Olive oil
- Paprika
- Pure vanilla extract
- Protein powder
- Red pepper flakes
- Reduced-sodium soy sauce
- Rice vinegar
- Sesame oil
- Sesame seeds
- Sriracha
- Vanilla granola
- Vinaigrette (or prep Classic Vinaigrette on p.50)
- Walnuts

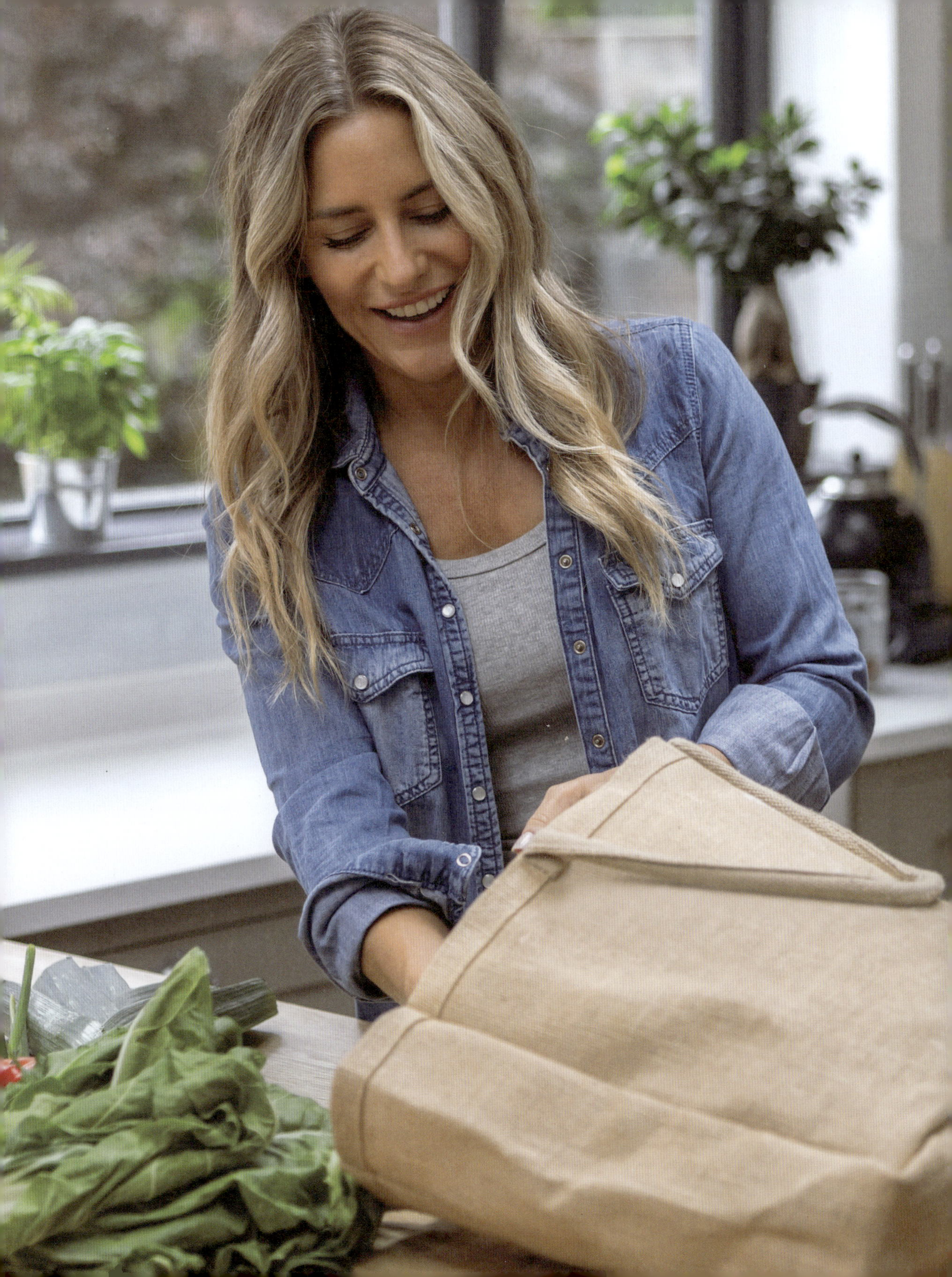

Day 1

BREAKFAST
Cheesy Avocado Omelet + ¾ cup vanilla Greek yogurt with ¼ cup each blueberries and vanilla granola

SNACK
Apple Energy Balls (3 pieces) 🥡

LUNCH
White Bean, Tuna, and Roasted Pepper Salad

SNACK
⅓ cup prepared hummus + 8 baby carrots 🔪

DINNER
Parmesan Chicken & Roasted Tomato Sandwich + Quick Roasted Broccoli

Day 2 - FASTING

LUNCH
Southwestern Chopped Salad + Avocado Toast 🔪

SNACK
Berry, Chia, and Mint Smoothie 🔪

SNACK
15 almonds and 2 dark chocolate squares

DINNER
Smoky Chicken Thighs on Baby Romaine

Day 3

BREAKFAST
Blueberry Smoothie Bowl

SNACK
1 slice toasted whole-grain bread + 2 hard-boiled eggs sprinkled with Everything Bagel seasoning 🔪

LUNCH
White Bean, Tuna, and Roasted Pepper Salad 🥄 + Apple with 1 Tbsp almond butter (or your choice of nut butter)

SNACK
½ cup raspberries, part-skim cheese stick, and 1 oz almonds (approx. 20–22 pieces)

DINNER
Parmesan Chicken & Roasted Tomato Sandwich 🥄 + Lemony Green Beans

Day 4 - FASTING

LUNCH
Greek Turkey Burger + ⅓ cup prepared hummus and 8 baby carrots 🔪

SNACK
¾ cup Greek yogurt, ¼ cup vanilla granola, and 5 sliced strawberries

SNACK
Everything Bagel Salmon Breakfast Wrap (1 serving)

DINNER
Rainbow Chicken Slaw

Day 5

BREAKFAST
Oatmeal with Yogurt and Toasted Almonds

SNACK
Berry, Chia, and Mint Smoothie (2 servings)

LUNCH
Southwestern Chopped Salad 🥄 + 1 (5-oz) can tuna packed in water, drained (alternative: ½ cup shredded rotisserie chicken breast)

SNACK
Apple with 1 Tbsp almond butter (or your choice of nut butter)

DINNER
Tortellini and Pesto Snow Peas + Lemony Green Beans 🥄

Day 6 - FASTING

LUNCH
Rainbow Chicken Slaw 🥄 + 1 slice lavash flatbread, warmed

SNACK
Blueberry Smoothie Bowl

SNACK
½ cup sliced strawberries, 1 oz almonds (approximately 20–22 pieces), and 1 dark chocolate square

DINNER
Tortellini and Pesto Snow Peas 🥄 + Simple side salad

Day 7

BREAKFAST
Everything Bagel Salmon Breakfast Wrap 🥄 + ½ cup raspberries

SNACK
Apple Energy Balls (3 pieces) 🥡 + ¾ cup Greek yogurt

LUNCH
Shrimp, Avocado, and Egg Chopped Salad 🔪

SNACK
1 slice toasted whole-grain bread topped with 2 Tbsp almond butter (or your choice of nut butter)

DINNER
Greek Turkey Burger + Quick Roasted Broccoli

🥡 **Fully prepped**

🔪 **Partially prepped**

🥄 **Leftover**

SHOPPING LIST

PRODUCE

1	small red onion
⅛	sweet onion
3	cremini mushrooms
½	cup baby spinach
2	cups grape tomatoes
½	pt cherry tomatoes
½	tomato
4	Tbsp parsley
3	avocados
¾	cup blueberries
½	cup dried apples
2	apples
3	pitted Medjool dates
1	large romaine heart
2½	heads romaine lettuce
1	cup shredded romaine lettuce
1	shallot
16	baby carrots
2	small carrots
2½	cups arugula
3	cups broccoli florets
½	cup cilantro
2	limes
2	Persian cucumbers
1	small red bell pepper
3	cups strawberries
2	cups raspberries
4	beets
1	cup mint leaves
3	lemons
2	cups green beans
3	scallions
3	cloves garlic
1	small zucchini

MEAT & SEAFOOD

3	thin chicken cutlets
6	oz large shrimp
12	large peeled and deveined shrimp
2	5-oz boneless, skinless chicken thighs
1	lb lean ground white-meat turkey
3	oz sliced smoked salmon
1½	cups shredded rotisserie chicken

REFRIGERATOR & DAIRY

8	eggs
1	oz Cheddar
4	Tbsp grated Parmesan
1	part-skim cheese stick
1	oz feta cheese
½	lb fresh cheese tortellini
1½	cups vanilla low-fat Greek yogurt
1⅓	cups plain fat-free Greek yogurt

⅔	cup hummus
2½	cups unsweetened almond milk
½	cup buttermilk
¼	cup orange juice

FROZEN

1	cup frozen blueberries

BREAD & BAKERY

½	cup vanilla granola
½	baguette
1	corn tortilla
3	slices whole-grain bread
2	whole-wheat buns
3	lavash flatbread
1½	slices sourdough bread

PANTRY

1¼	cup extra-virgin olive oil
1	Tbsp basil pesto
½	Tbsp honey
1¼	tsp ground cinnamon
⅛	tsp ground nutmeg
¾	cup cannellini beans
1	jarred roasted red pepper
¼	cup marinated artichoke hearts
¼	cup pitted mixed olives

½	5-oz can tuna packed in olive oil
1	5-oz can tuna packed in water
⅓	cup red wine vinegar
1	Tbsp Dijon mustard
2	tsp honey mustard
½	tsp garlic powder
¾	cup low-sodium black beans
¼	tsp paprika
1	tsp smoked paprika
3⅓	Tbsp Everything Bagel seasoning
2	Tbsp chia seeds
3	oz dry-roasted almonds
3½	Tbsp sliced almonds
3	pieces dark chocolate squares
1	jarred pepperoncini peppers
1½	scoop protein powder
1	tsp vanilla extract
2	tsp hemp seeds
4	Tbsp almond butter or other nut butter
½	tsp ground cumin
¼	cup quick-cooking steel-cut oats
2	cups low-sodium vegetable or chicken broth

MEAL PREP DAY

Make it easy by partially prepping the day before you start your week.

APPLE ENERGY BALLS (P. 49)

FREEZE 2 SERVINGS BERRY, CHIA, MINT, AND BEETS

For Berry, Chia, and Mint Smoothie (p. 57) on Days 2 and 5

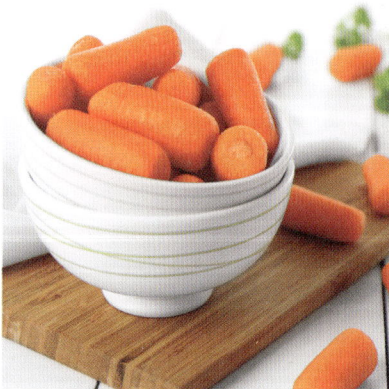

BABY CARROTS

Portion out what you need in Ziploc bags for Days 1 and 4

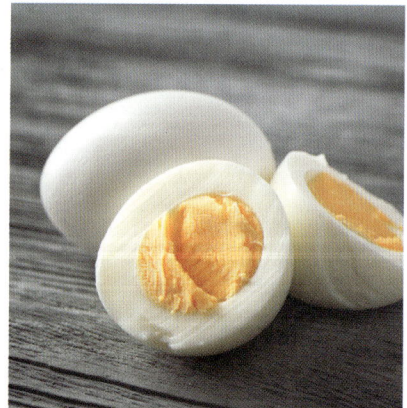

4 HARD-BOILED EGGS

For Shrimp, Avocado, and Egg Chopped Salad (p. 73), lunch on Day 2, and snack on Day 3

MEAL PLAN
DAY 1

BREAKFAST
Cheesy Avocado
Omelet (p. 46) + ¾ cup
vanilla Greek yogurt
with ¼ cup each
blueberries and vanilla
granola

SNACK
Apple Energy Balls
(3 pieces) ⬜ (p. 49)

LUNCH
White Bean, Tuna, and
Roasted Pepper Salad
(p. 50)

SNACK
⅓ cup prepared
hummus + 8 baby
carrots ✎

DINNER
Parmesan Chicken
& Roasted Tomato
Sandwich (p. 53) + Quick
Roasted Broccoli: Toss
1½ cups broccoli florets
with 1 Tbsp olive oil and
⅛ tsp garlic powder.
Bake at 400°F for 9 to 11
min. or until edges are
starting to brown.

WATER

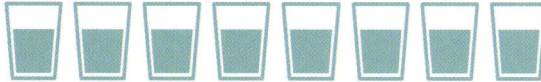

MOVEMENT Y ☐ N ☐

ACTIVITY	DURATION	INTENSITY

SLEEP

BEDTIME	WAKE UP

MOOD

☺ ☺ ☹

39

MEAL PLAN
DAY 2

LUNCH
Southwestern Chopped Salad (p. 54) + Avocado Toast 🔪: Spread ⅓ cup mashed avocado over a toasted slice of whole-grain bread. Top with a sliced hard boiled egg and sprinkle with Everything Bagel seasoning.

SNACK
Berry, Chia, and Mint Smoothie 🔪 (p. 57)

SNACK
15 almonds and 2 dark chocolate squares

DINNER
Smoky Chicken Thighs on Baby Romaine (p. 58)

WATER

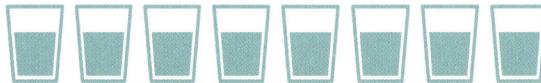

MOVEMENT Y ☐ N ☐

ACTIVITY	DURATION	INTENSITY

SLEEP

BEDTIME	WAKE UP

MOOD

🙂 😐 🙁

MEAL PLAN
DAY 3

BREAKFAST
Blueberry Smoothie
Bowl (p. 61)

SNACK
1 slice toasted whole-
grain bread + 2 hard-
boiled eggs sprinkled
with Everything Bagel
seasoning 🖊

LUNCH
White Bean, Tuna, and
Roasted Pepper Salad
🍵 + Apple with 1 Tbsp
almond butter (or your
choice of nut butter)

SNACK
½ cup raspberries,
part-skim cheese stick,
and 1 oz almonds
(approximately 20 to 22
pieces)

DINNER
Parmesan Chicken
& Roasted Tomato
Sandwich 🍵 + Lemony
Green Beans: Toss
2 cups steamed green
beans with 4 tsp olive oil
or butter and 1½ to
2 tsp lemon juice.
Reserve half for Day 5
dinner.

WATER

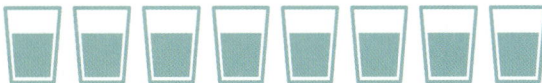

MOVEMENT Y ☐ N ☐

ACTIVITY	DURATION	INTENSITY

SLEEP

BEDTIME	WAKE UP

MOOD

☺ ☻ ☹

MEAL PLAN
DAY 4

LUNCH
Greek Turkey Burger
(p. 62) + ⅓ cup prepared
hummus & 8 baby
carrots

SNACK
¾ cup Greek yogurt,
¼ cup vanilla
granola, and 5 sliced
strawberries

SNACK
Everything Bagel
Salmon Breakfast
Wrap (p. 65)

DINNER
Rainbow Chicken
Slaw (p. 66)

WATER

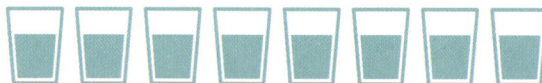

MOVEMENT Y ☐ N ☐

ACTIVITY	DURATION	INTENSITY

SLEEP

BEDTIME	WAKE UP

MOOD

☺ ☺ ☹

MEAL PLAN
DAY 5

BREAKFAST
Oatmeal with Yogurt
and Toasted Almonds
(p. 69)

SNACK
Berry, Chia, and Mint
Smoothie (p. 57)

LUNCH
Southwestern Chopped
Salad ♻ + 1 (5-oz) can
tuna packed in water,
drained (alternative:
½ cup shredded
rotisserie chicken
breast)

SNACK
Apple with 1 Tbsp
almond butter (or your
choice of nut butter)

DINNER
Tortellini and Pesto
Snow Peas (p. 70) +
Lemony Green Beans ♻

WATER

MOVEMENT Y ☐ N ☐

ACTIVITY	DURATION	INTENSITY

SLEEP

BEDTIME	WAKE UP

MOOD

MEAL PLAN
DAY 6

LUNCH
Rainbow Chicken Slaw ♨ + 1 slice lavash flatbread, warmed

SNACK
Blueberry Smoothie Bowl (p. 61)

SNACK
½ cup sliced strawberries, 1 oz almonds (approximately 20 to 22 pieces), and 1 dark chocolate square

DINNER
Tortellini and Pesto Snow Peas ♨ + Simple side salad: Toss 1½ cup arugula or other leafy greens with 2 Tbsp vinaigrette.

WATER

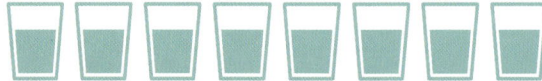

MOVEMENT Y ☐ N ☐

ACTIVITY	DURATION	INTENSITY

SLEEP

BEDTIME	WAKE UP

MOOD

☺ 😐 ☹

MEAL PLAN
DAY 7

BREAKFAST
Everything Bagel
Salmon Breakfast Wrap
🍲 + ½ cup raspberries

SNACK
Apple Energy Balls
(3 pieces) 🍽 + ¾ cup
Greek yogurt

LUNCH
Shrimp, Avocado, and
Egg Chopped Salad ✐
(p. 73)

SNACK
1 slice toasted whole-
grain bread topped with
2 Tbsp almond butter
(or your choice of nut
butter)

DINNER
Greek Turkey Burger 🍲 +
Quick Roasted Broccoli:
Toss 1½ cups broccoli
florets with 1 Tbsp olive
oil and ⅛ tsp garlic
powder. Bake at 400°F
for 9 to 11 min. or
until edges are starting
to brown.

WATER

MOVEMENT Y ☐ N ☐

ACTIVITY	DURATION	INTENSITY

SLEEP

BEDTIME	WAKE UP

MOOD

🙂 😐 ☹️

CHEESY AVOCADO OMELET

ACTIVE **5 MIN.**
TOTAL **15 MIN.**
SERVES **1**

1	tsp olive oil
½	small red onion, finely chopped
	Kosher salt and pepper
3	cremini mushrooms, sliced
½	cup baby spinach
2	large eggs plus 1 egg whites
1	oz sharp Cheddar, coarsely grated
½	cup grape tomatoes, halved
⅛	cup flat-leaf parsley, chopped
¼	small avocado

DIRECTIONS

1. In a medium nonstick skillet, heat oil on medium. Add onion, season with pinch each salt and pepper and cook, stirring occasionally for 4 min. Add mushrooms and cook, stirring occasionally until just tender, 4 min. Stir in spinach and cook until beginning to wilt.

2. Add eggs and cook, stirring for 1 min., then cook without stirring until edges are brown, 2 to 3 min. Sprinkle with cheese and fold one half over the other to create a semicircle.

3. Toss tomatoes with parsley and avocado and serve spooned over omelet.

NUTRITION
PER SERVING 350 cal, 32 g pro, 10 g carb, 10 g fiber, 7 g sugars (0 g added sugars), 22 g fat (8 g sat fat), 200 mg chol, 300 mg sodium

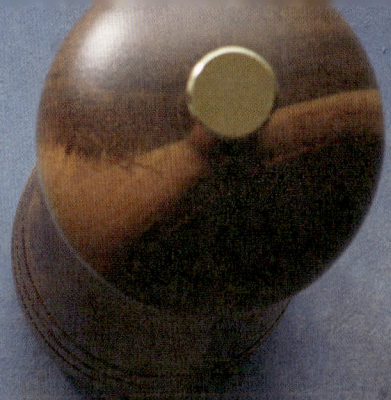

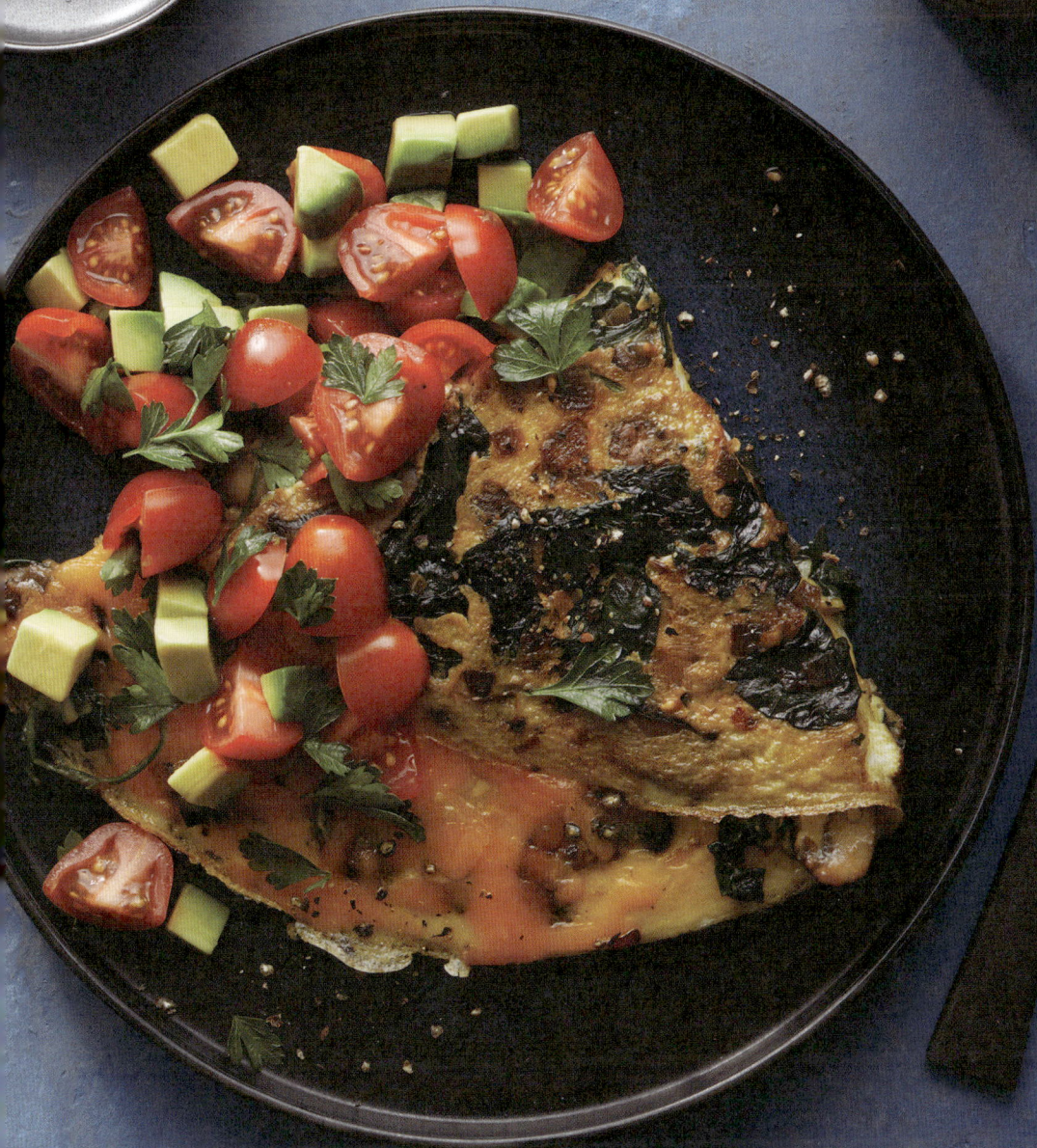

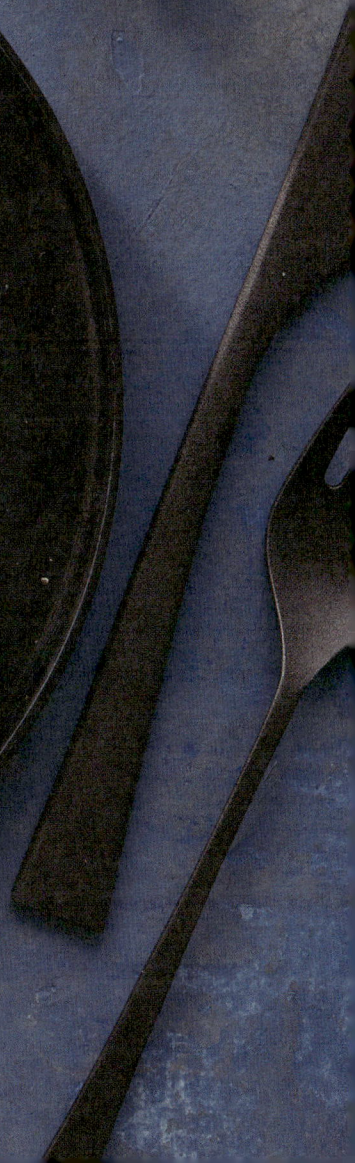

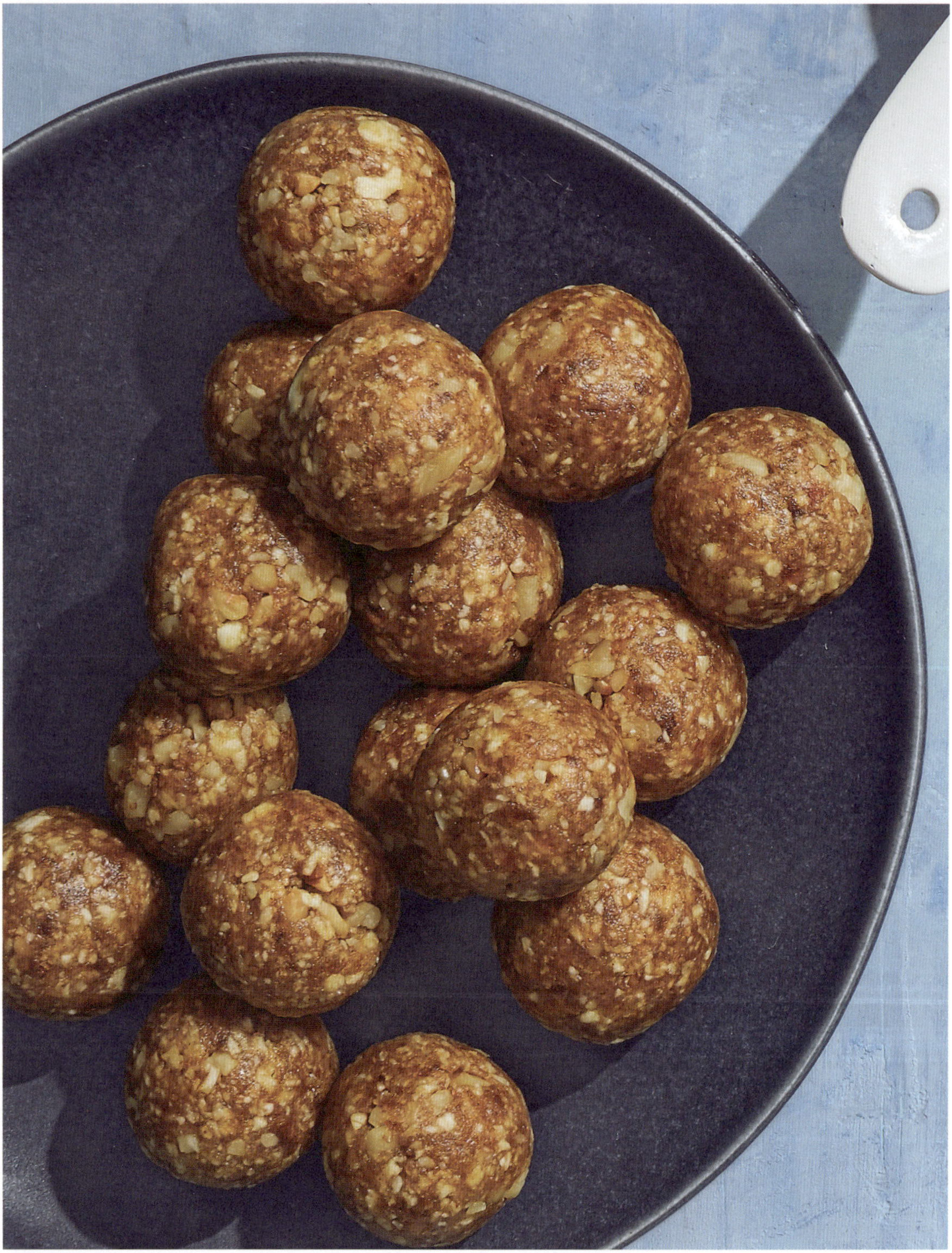

APPLE ENERGY BALLS

ACTIVE **20 MIN.**
TOTAL **2 HR 10 MIN.**
SERVES **6**

½   cup dried apples, chopped
3   pitted Medjool dates
½   Tbsp honey
¼   tsp ground cinnamon
⅛   tsp freshly ground nutmeg
     Kosher salt
¼   cup toasted walnuts

DIRECTIONS

1. In a food processor, puree apples, dates, honey, cinnamon, nutmeg, and a pinch of salt until almost smooth. Add walnuts and pulse to incorporate.

2. Firmly roll into 1-in. balls. Refrigerate at least 2 hours and up to 5 days.

NUTRITION
PER BALL 75 cal, 1 g pro, 14 g carb, 2 g fiber, 11.5 g sugars (1.5 g added sugars), 2.5 g fat (0.5 g sat fat), 0 mg chol, 15 mg sodium

WHITE BEAN, TUNA, AND ROASTED PEPPER SALAD

ACTIVE **10 MIN.**
TOTAL **40 MIN.**
SERVES **1**

¾   cup cannellini beans, rinsed

¼   small red onion, finely chopped

3   Tbsp vinaigrette

1   large romaine heart, torn into pieces

1   jarred roasted red pepper, drained and cut into pieces

¼   cup marinated artichoke hearts, drained and quartered

¼   cup pitted mixed olives

½   5-oz can tuna packed in olive oil, drained and flaked

DIRECTIONS

In a large bowl, toss beans and onion with vinaigrette, then add lettuce and toss to coat. Fold in pepper, artichoke hearts, olives, and tuna.

NUTRITION

PER SERVING 310 cal, 15 g pro, 25 g carb, 11 g fiber, 2 g sugars (0 g added sugars), 17 g fat (3 g sat fat), 13 mg chol, 815 mg sodium

CLASSIC VINAIGRETTE

ACTIVE **5 MIN.**
TOTAL **5 MIN.**
MAKES **ABOUT 1 CUP**

DIRECTIONS

To a jar, add ⅓ cup **red wine vinegar**, 1 **shallot** (finely chopped), 1 Tbsp **Dijon mustard**, ½ tsp **kosher salt**, and ¼ tsp **pepper**. Cover and shake to combine. Add ½ cup **extra-virgin olive oil**. Cover and shake until emulsified. Dressing will keep in fridge for up to 5 days.

NUTRITION

PER TABLESPOON 65 cal, 0 g pro, 0 g carb, 0 g fiber, 0g sugars (0 g added sugars), 7 g fat (1 g sat fat), 0 mg chol, 85 mg sodium

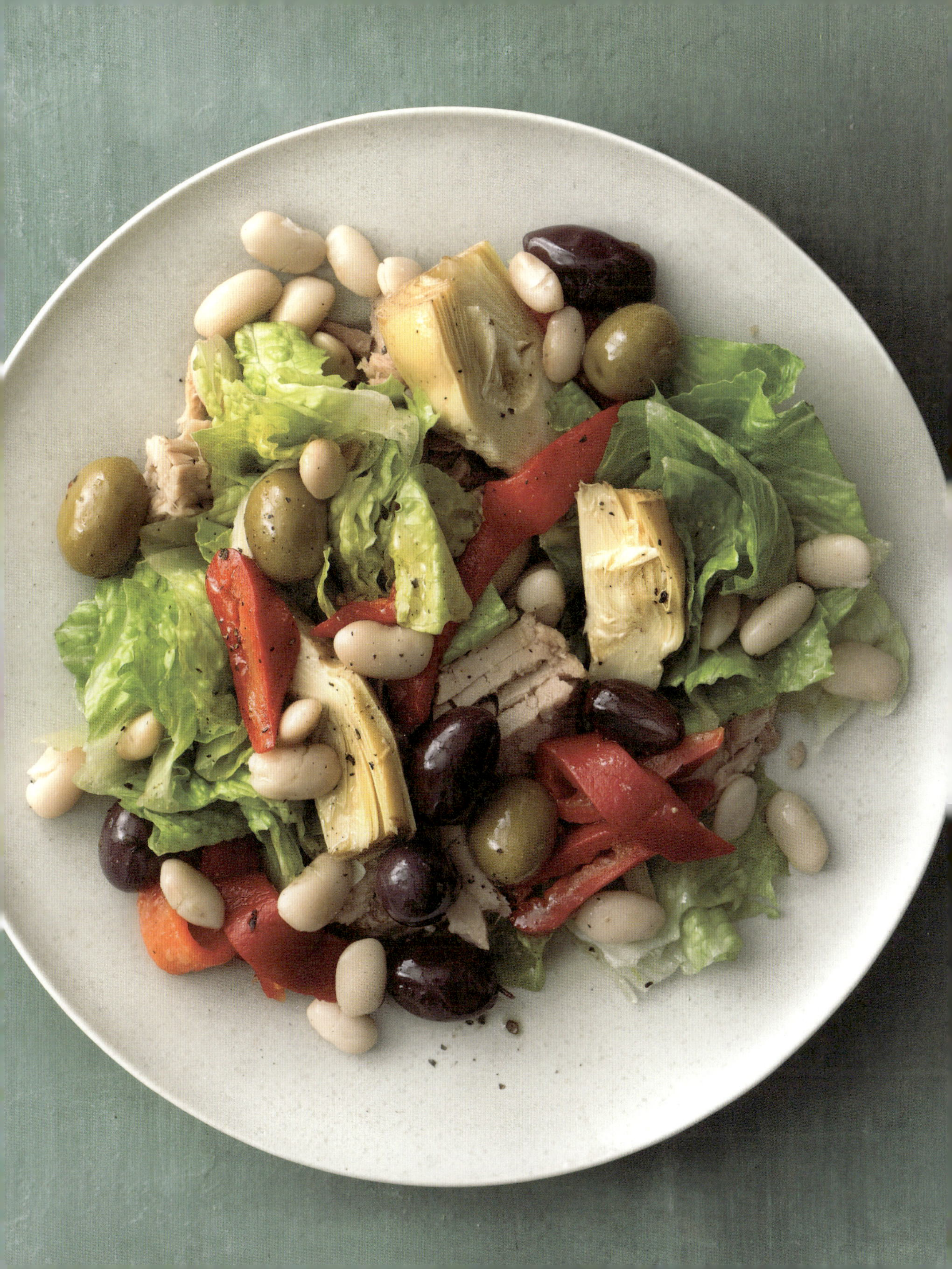

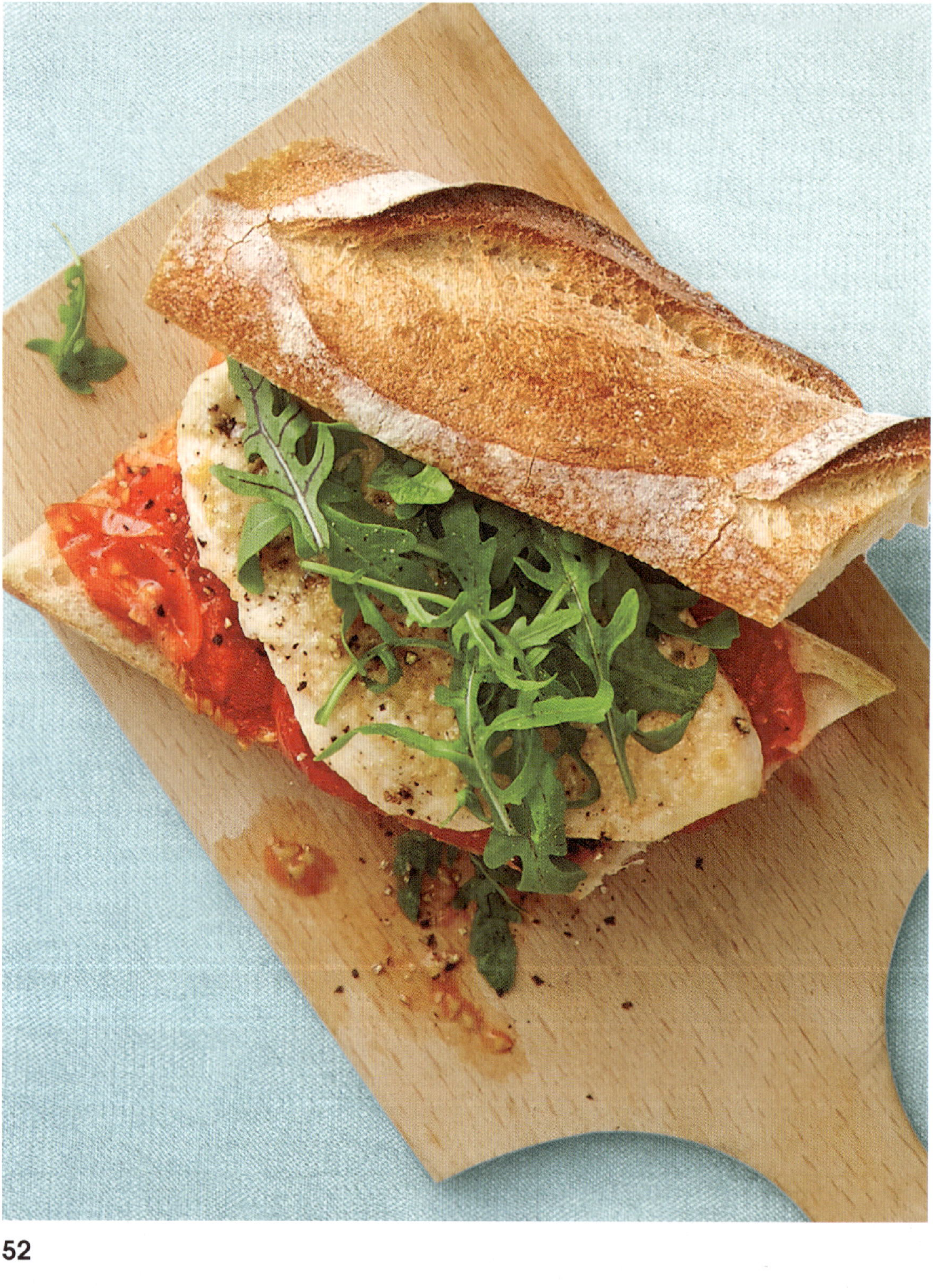

PARMESAN CHICKEN AND ROASTED TOMATO SANDWICHES

ACTIVE **10 MIN.**
TOTAL **20 MIN.**
SERVES **2**

3	small, thin chicken cutlets
1½	Tbsp olive oil, divided
¼	tsp garlic powder
	Kosher salt and pepper
1	Tbsp grated Parmesan
1	cup grape tomatoes
½	baguette, halved
1	cup arugula, divided

DIRECTIONS

1. Heat oven to 450°F and line a broiler proof pan with foil. Place chicken on one side of pan. Brush tops of chicken cutlets with 1 tsp olive oil, then season with garlic powder and ¼ tsp each salt and pepper and sprinkle with 1 Tbsp grated Parmesan.

2. Place tomatoes on the other side and drizzle with remaining ½ Tbsp olive oil and roast 6 min., then broil until golden brown and cooked through, about 2 min.

3. Split half baguette and smash half tomatoes on the bottom split half, then top with half chicken and ½ cup arugula. Refrigerate remaining chicken, tomatoes, and arugula separately to make a second sandwich later in the week.

NUTRITION
PER SERVING 375 cal, 40 g pro, 29 g carb, 4 g fiber, 2 g sugars (0 g added sugars), 10 g fat (2 g sat fat), 95 mg chol, 610 mg sodium

SOUTHWESTERN CHOPPED SALAD

ACTIVE **10 MIN.**
TOTAL **20 MIN.**
SERVES **2**

SALAD

1	corn tortilla
¼	avocado
1	Tbsp fat-free Greek yogurt
¼	cup cilantro
2	Tbsp fresh lime juice
2	Tbsp water
½	head romaine lettuce, chopped
¾	cup low-sodium black beans, rinsed
2	Persian cucumbers, sliced
1	small red pepper, sliced

SHRIMP

½	Tbsp olive oil
12	large peeled and deveined shrimp
½	tsp paprika
	Kosher salt and pepper

DIRECTIONS

1. Heat oven to 400°F. Place sliced tortillas on a baking sheet and roast until crisp.

2. In a mini blender, puree avocado, Greek yogurt, cilantro, lime juice, and water.

3. Toss dressing with romaine lettuce, then fold in black beans, cucumber, and red pepper.

4. Heat oil in a medium skillet on medium-high. Season shrimp with paprika and pinch each salt and pepper, and cook until opaque throughout, about 2 min. per side.

5. Top salad with shrimp and tortilla strips.

NUTRITION

PER SERVING 295 cal, 27 g pro, 31 g carb, 13 g fiber, 4 g sugars (0 g added sugars), 9 g fat (1 g sat fat), 136 mg chol, 435 mg sodium

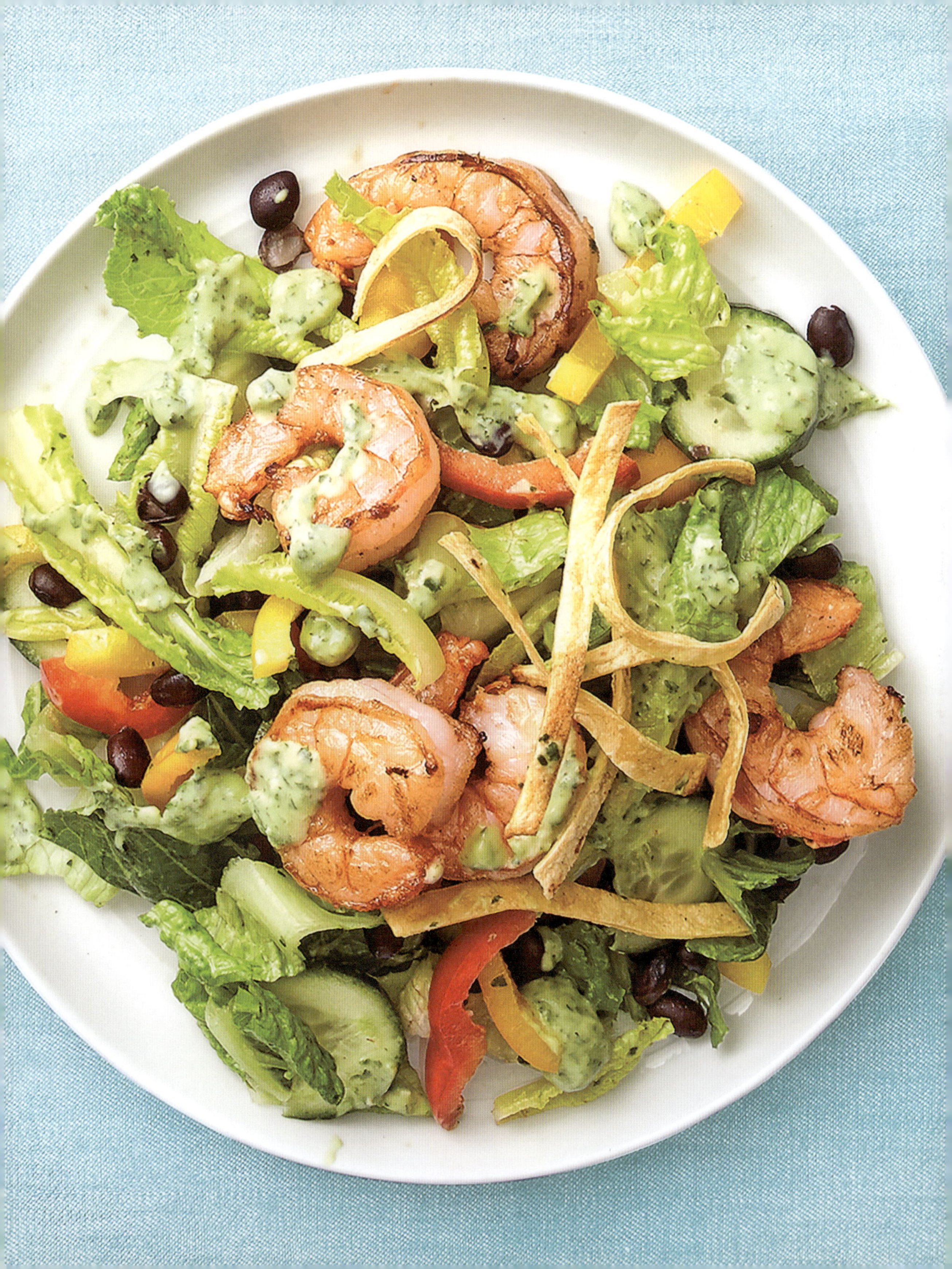

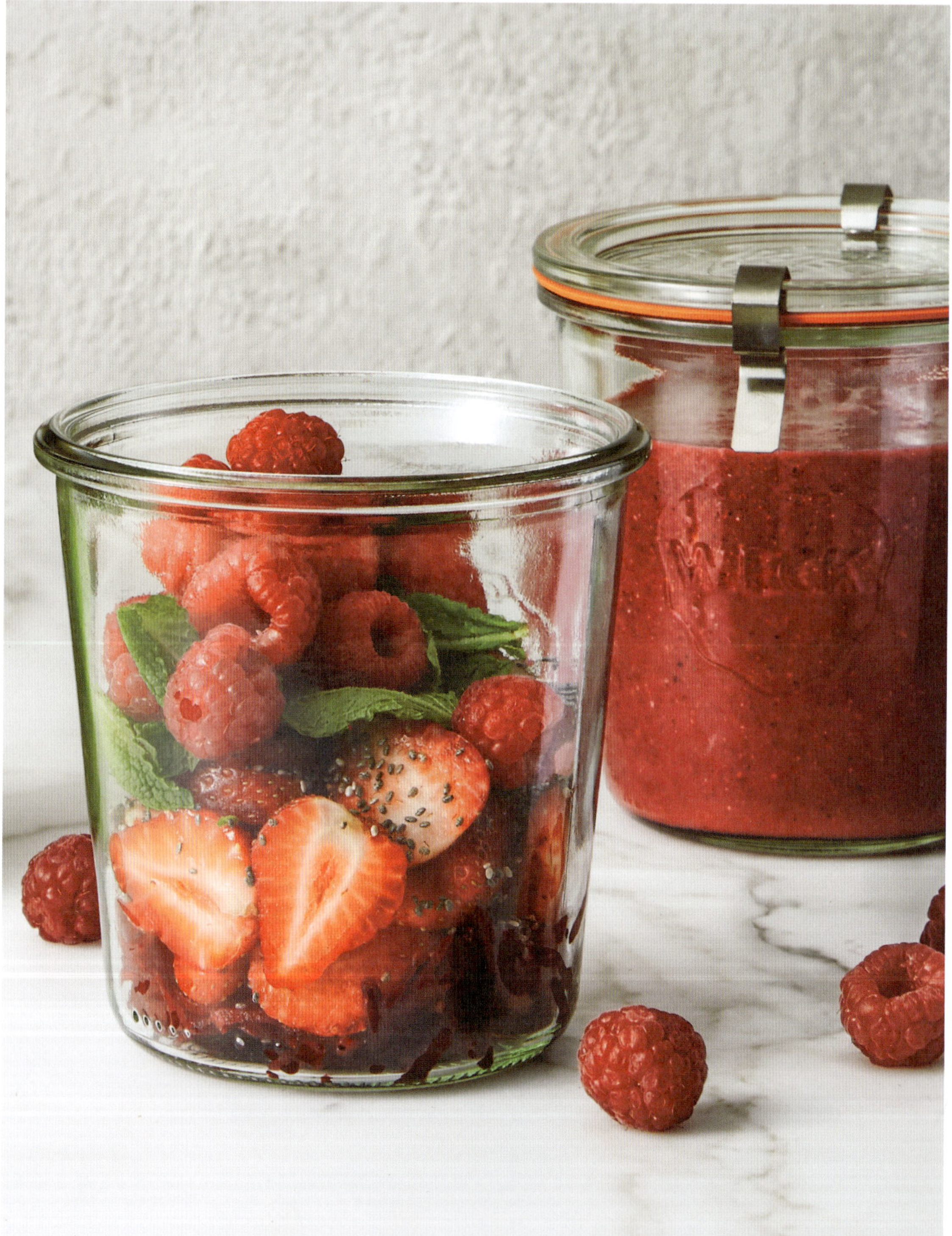
WECK

BERRY, CHIA, AND MINT SMOOTHIE

ACTIVE **10 MIN.**
TOTAL **40 MIN.**
SERVES **1**

1	cup sliced strawberries
½	cup raspberries
½	cup grated beet (from 1 medium beet)
⅓	cup mint leaves
2	Tbsp chia seeds
1	cup unsweetened almond milk

DIRECTIONS

1. Place berries, beet, mint, and chia seeds in resealable plastic bag or freezer-safe jar. Freeze overnight or longer.

2. When ready to prepare, add almond milk to blender, then add frozen ingredients. Blend until smooth.

NUTRITION
PER SERVING 210 cal, 6 g pro, 34 g carb, 16 g fiber, 14 g sugars (0 g added sugars), 7 g fat (1 g sat fat), 0 mg chol, 25 mg sodium

SMOKY CHICKEN THIGHS ON BABY ROMAINE

ACTIVE **20 MIN.**
TOTAL **20 MIN.**
SERVES **2**

2½	Tbsp fresh lemon juice
2½	Tbsp plus 1 tsp olive oil, divided
1½	large cloves garlic, grated
1¾	tsp smoked paprika, divided
	Kosher salt
2	5-oz boneless, skinless chicken thighs
½	pint cherry tomatoes, halved
1	jarred pepperoncini pepper, sliced
⅛	cup flat-leaf parsley, chopped
1½	slices sourdough bread, toasted
2	heads baby romaine or Little Gem lettuce, halved or quartered if large)
½	avocado, cubed

DIRECTIONS

1. In a medium bowl, whisk together lemon juice, ⅓ cup olive oil, garlic, 1½ tsp smoked paprika, and ½ tsp salt.

2. Transfer 1 cup of dressing to a resealable bag, add chicken thighs, and marinate 30 min. to 2 hr.; reserve remaining dressing.

3. Heat 1 tsp olive oil in a large skillet on medium. Season chicken with ¼ tsp salt and cook until golden brown, 4 to 5 min. per side. Transfer to cutting board, sprinkle with ¼ tsp smoked paprika, and slice.

4. In reserved dressing, toss cherry tomatoes, pepperoncini pepper, and parsley. Tear sourdough bread into bite-size pieces and scatter over baby romaine or Little Gem lettuce. Top with tomato mixture, avocado, and chicken.

NUTRITION
PER SERVING 555 cal, 32 g pro, 34 g carb, 7 g fiber, 5 g sugars (0 g added sugars), 33 g fat (6 g sat fat), 130 mg chol, 810 mg sodium

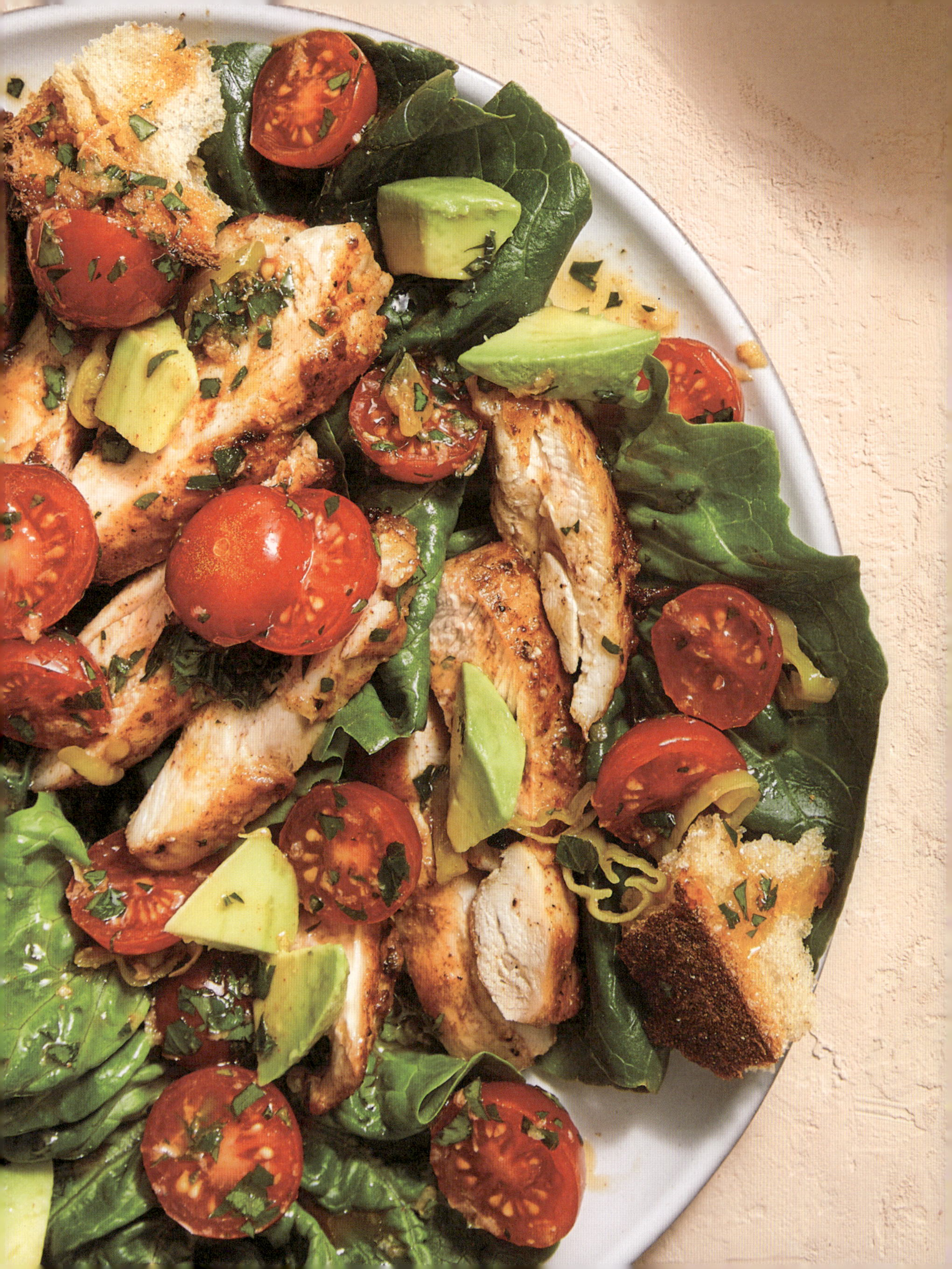

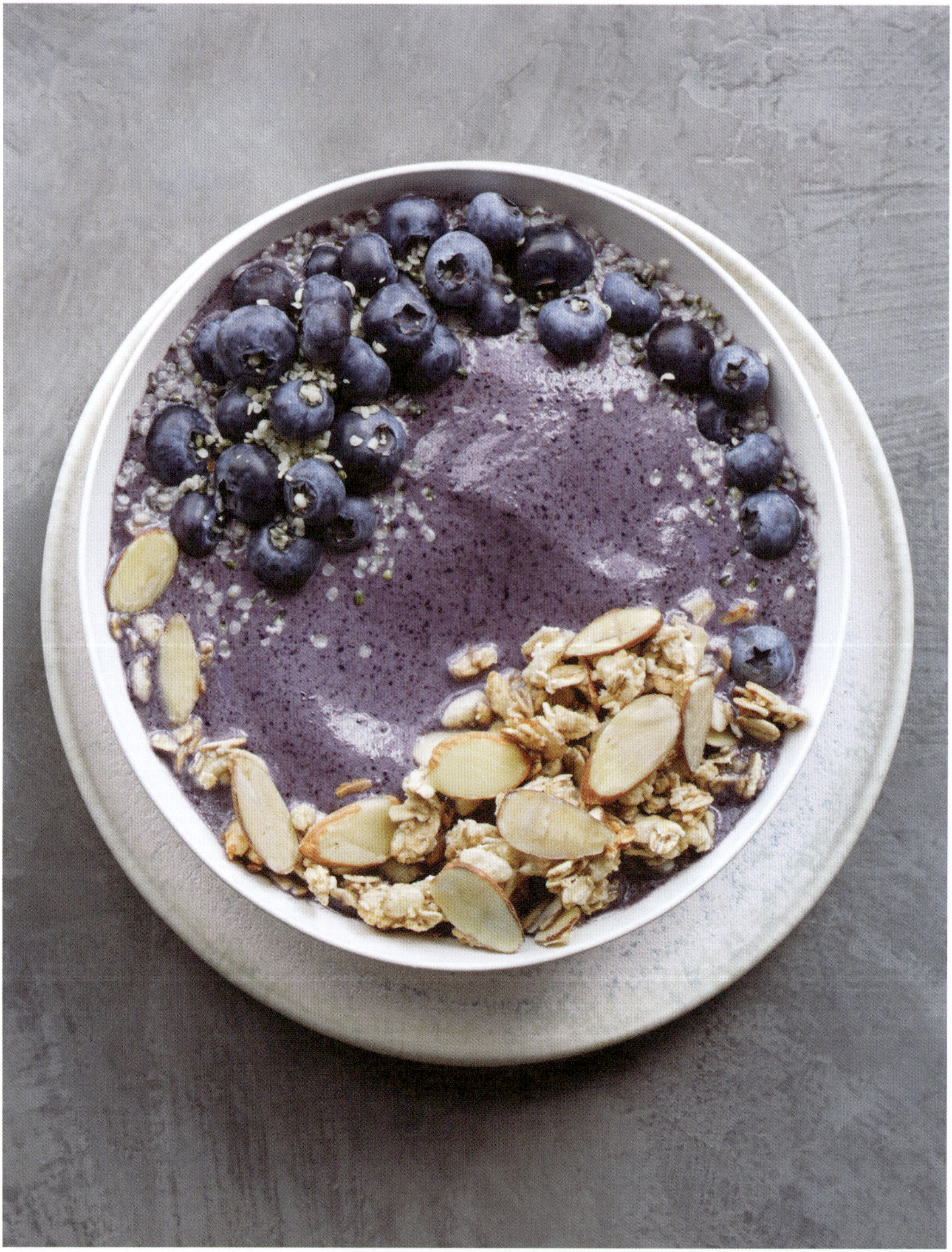

BLUEBERRY SMOOTHIE BOWL

ACTIVE **10 MIN.**
TOTAL **10 MIN.**
SERVES **1**

½	**cup frozen blueberries**
¼	**cup unsweetened almond milk**
¾	**scoop protein powder**
1	**Tbsp unsweetened almond butter**
½	**tsp pure vanilla extract**
¼	**cup fresh blueberries**
⅛	**cup vanilla granola**
1	**Tbsp sliced almonds**
1	**tsp hemp seeds**
½	**tsp ground cinnamon**

DIRECTIONS

1. In a blender, puree frozen blueberries, almond milk, protein powder, almond butter, and vanilla until creamy. Divide between two bowls.

2. Top each bowl with fresh blueberries, granola, almonds, hemp seeds, and cinnamon before serving.

NUTRITION
PER SERVING 370 cal, 25 g pro, 32 g carb, 7 g fiber, 16 g sugars (4 g added sugars), 17 g fat (2.5 g sat fat), 0 mg chol, 130 mg sodium

GREEK TURKEY BURGERS

ACTIVE **10 MIN.**
TOTAL **20 MIN.**
SERVES **2**

1	lb lean ground white-meat turkey
2	scallions, finely chopped
1	clove garlic, finely chopped
1	small zucchini, grated
1	large egg white
¼	cup fresh mint, sliced
½	tsp ground cumin
	Kosher salt and pepper
3	tsp olive oil, divided
½	tomato, chopped
⅛	sweet onion, finely chopped
½	oz feta cheese
	Lettuce and whole-wheat buns, for serving

DIRECTIONS

1. Combine turkey, scallions, garlic, zucchini, egg white, mint, ground cumin, and 1/2 tsp each salt and pepper. Shape into four ½-in.-thick patties. Freeze half the patties to cook at another time.

2. Heat olive oil in a nonstick skillet on medium. Cook until burgers are done, about 5 min. per side.

3. Meanwhile, combine tomato, sweet onion, olive oil, and feta for tomato-feta relish.

4. Serve on whole-wheat buns with lettuce and tomato-feta relish.

NUTRITION
PER SERVING 380 cal, 28 g pro, 28 g carb, 5 g fiber, 5 g sugars (2 g added sugars), 17 g fat (4 g sat fat), 103 mg chol, 590 mg sodium

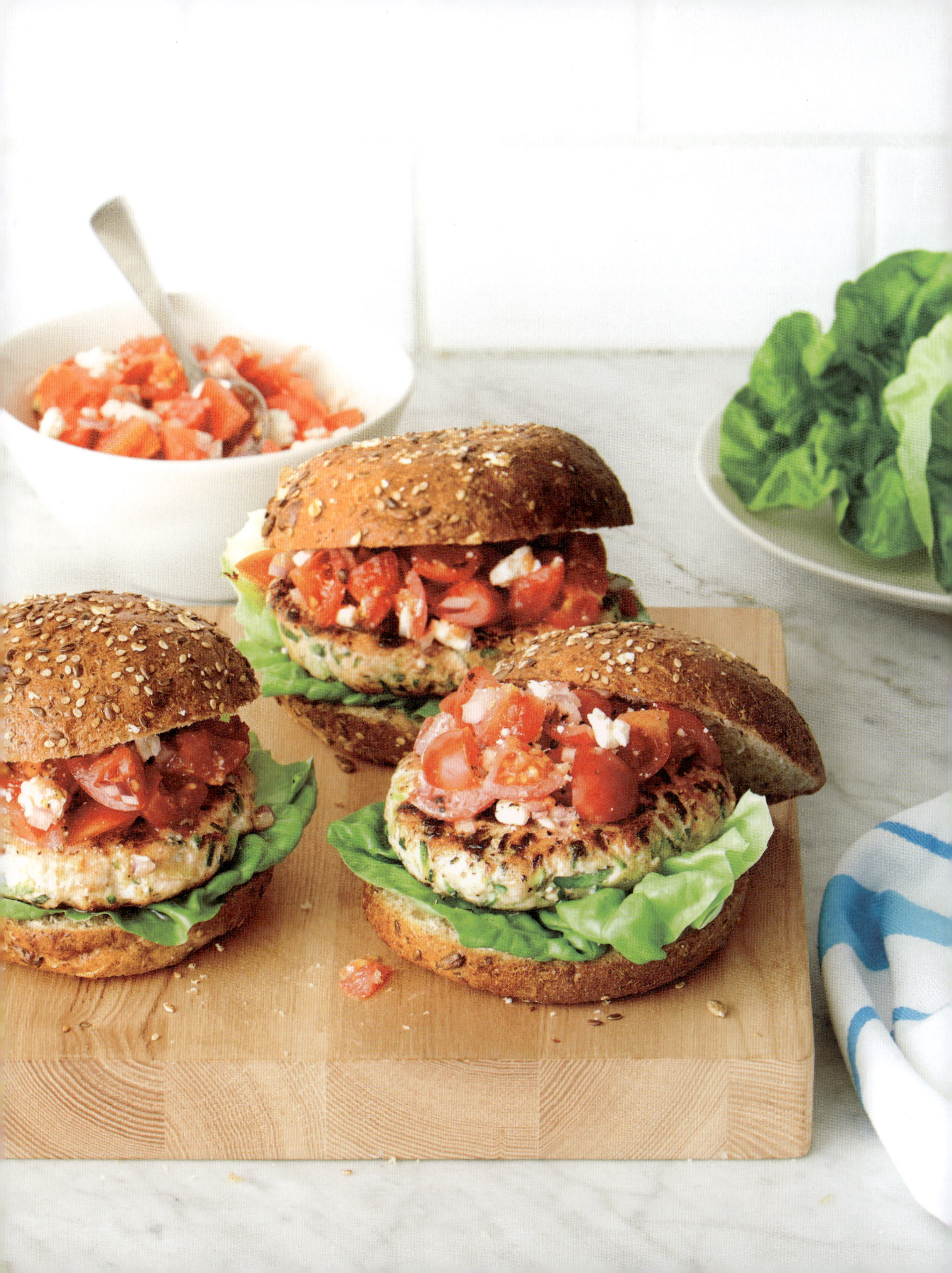

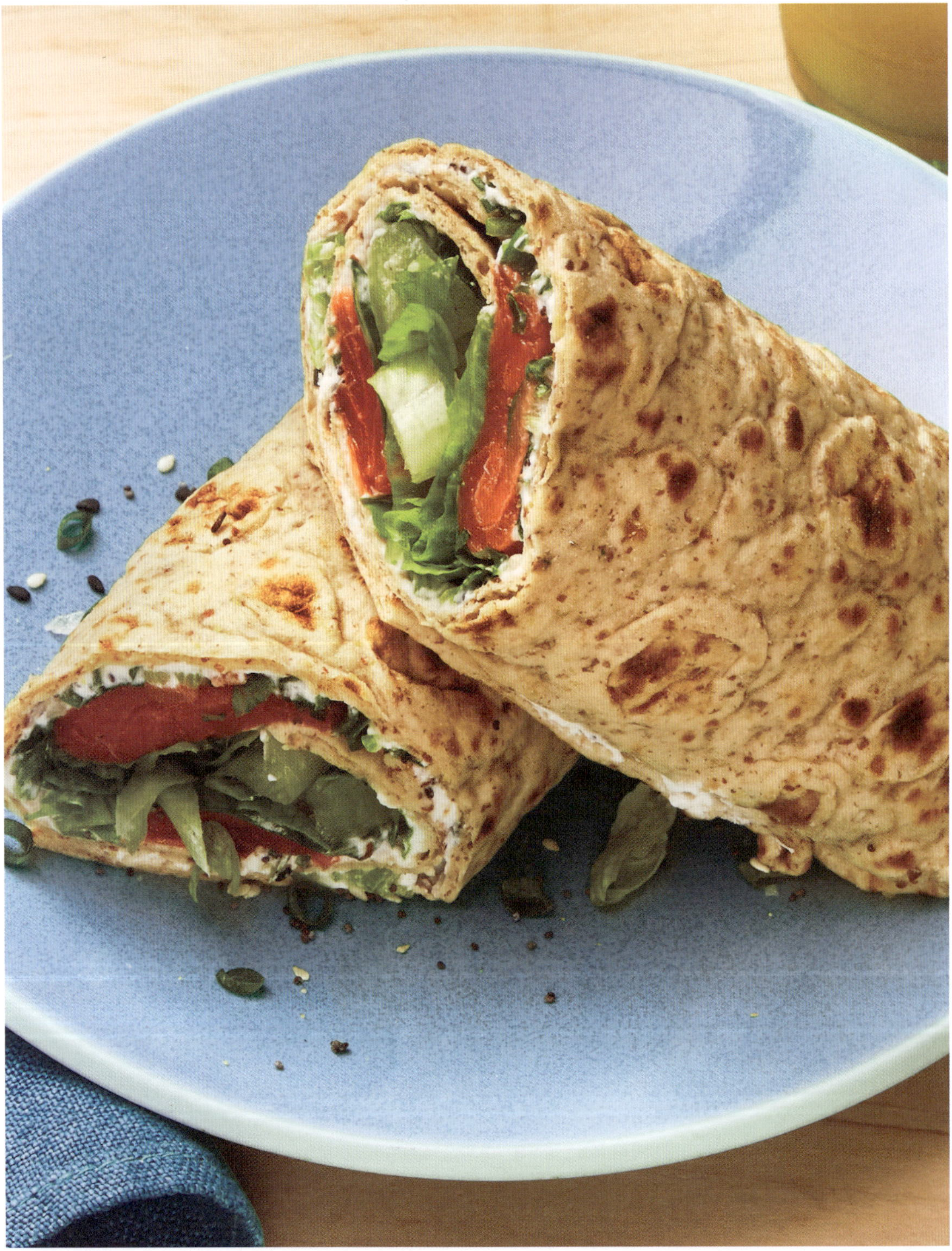

EVERYTHING BAGEL SALMON BREAKFAST WRAP

ACTIVE **10 MIN.**
TOTAL **10 MIN.**
SERVES **1**

1	lavash flatbread
3	Tbsp Greek yogurt
1½	Tbsp Everything Bagel seasoning mix
1	scallion, thinly sliced
1½	oz sliced smoked salmon
	Black pepper
½	cup shredded romaine lettuce

DIRECTIONS

1. Spread flatbread with yogurt, leaving a 1-in. border. Sprinkle with seasoning mix and scallion. Top with smoked salmon and season with ¼ tsp black pepper, then scatter shredded lettuce on top.

2. Fold in sides and roll up to enclose filling. Wrap in parchment or foil and refrigerate up to one day.

NUTRITION
PER SERVING 310 cal, 23 g pro, 41 g carb, 6 g fiber, 5 g sugars (2 g added sugars), 7 g fat (2 g sat fat), 16 mg chol, 650 mg sodium

RAINBOW CHICKEN SLAW

ACTIVE **20 MIN.**
TOTAL **20 MIN.**
SERVES **2**

½   cup buttermilk

4   tsp fresh lemon juice

2   cloves garlic, finely grated

2   tsp honey mustard

Kosher salt and pepper

1½ cups shredded cooked chicken

1   cup thinly sliced red cabbage

2   small carrots, coarsely grated

2   small rainbow or Chioggia beets, scrubbed and very thinly sliced

1   avocado, sliced

½   cup snow pea shoots

DIRECTIONS

1. In a medium bowl, whisk together buttermilk, lemon juice, garlic, honey mustard, and ¼ tsp pepper. Transfer half of dressing to a small bowl and set aside. Add chicken to remaining dressing in bowl and toss to coat.

2. Arrange cabbage, carrots, beets, avocado, and pea shoots on 2 large plates, drizzle with reserved dressing, and season with a pinch each of salt and pepper. Top with chicken.

NUTRITION

PER SERVING 460 cal, 32 g pro, 33 g carb, 12 g fiber, 16.5 g sugars (1.5 g added sugars), 24.5 g fat (4.5 g sat fat), 50 mg chol, 740 mg sodium

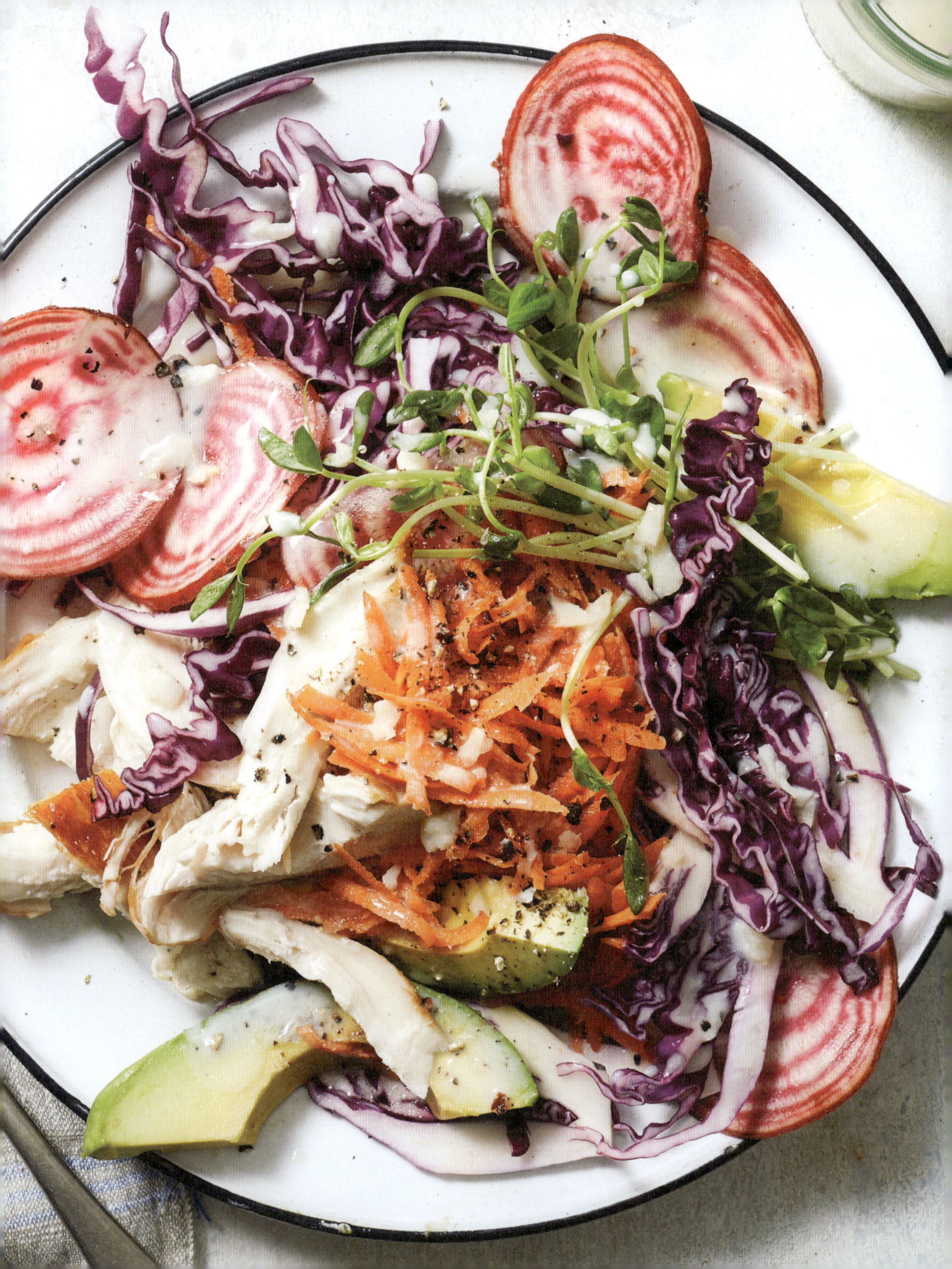

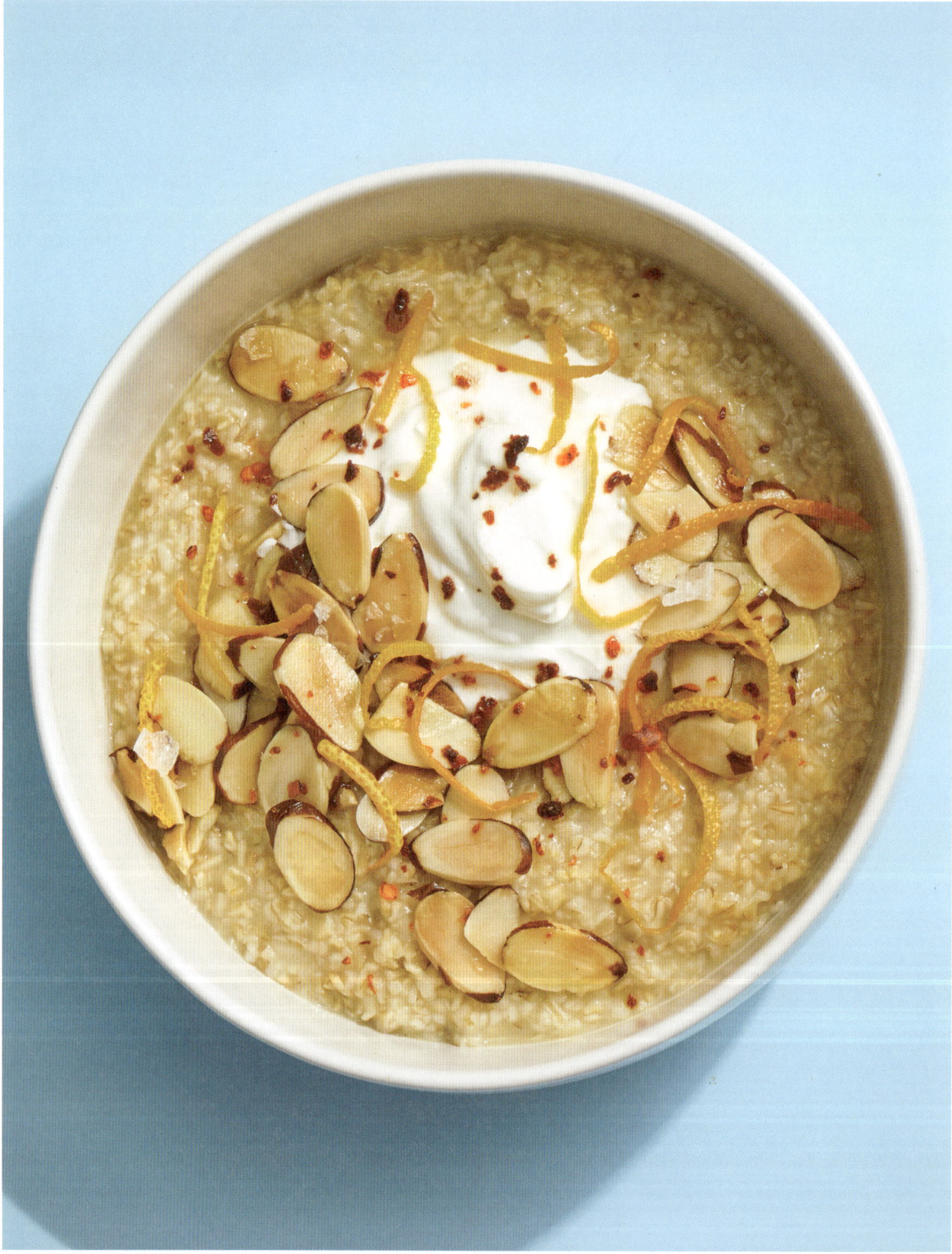

OATMEAL WITH YOGURT AND TOASTED ALMONDS

ACTIVE **10 MIN.**
TOTAL **10 MIN.**
SERVES **1**

½   cup water
¼   cup orange juice
¼   cup quick-cooking steel-cut oats
    Kosher salt
1½ Tbsp sliced almonds, toasted
1   tsp olive oil
2   Tbsp Greek yogurt
    Orange, for zesting
    Aleppo pepper and flaky salt, for serving

DIRECTIONS

1. In a small saucepan, bring water and orange juice to a boil. Add oats and pinch of salt and cook, stirring occasionally, until tender, 5 to 7 min.

2. In a small bowl, toss almonds with oil and pinch of salt.

3. Transfer oatmeal to serving bowl, top with yogurt and almonds, then grate orange zest over top and sprinkle with Aleppo pepper and flaky salt if desired.

NUTRITION
PER SERVING 340 cal, 10 g pro, 38 g carb, 5 g fiber, 10 g sugars (0 g added sugars), 17 g fat (3 g sat fat), 0 mg chol, 160 mg sodium

PESTO TORTELLINI AND SNOW PEAS

ACTIVE **20 MIN.**
TOTAL **20 MIN.**
SERVES **2**

2   cups low-sodium vegetable or chicken broth
½   lb fresh cheese tortellini
3   oz snow peas, strings removed, halved
1   Tbsp basil pesto
⅛   cup grated Parmesan, plus more for serving
     Zest of ½ lemon

DIRECTIONS

1. In a medium skillet, bring broth to a simmer. Add tortellini and simmer per package directions until barely tender, 4 to 5 min.

2. Stir in snow peas and simmer until tortellini and peas are tender, 1 to 2 min. Remove from heat and stir in pesto, then gently toss with Parmesan.

3. Working over skillet, finely grate in lemon zest. Serve with additional Parmesan if desired.

NUTRITION
PER SERVING 435 cal, 18 g pro, 61 g carb, 4 g fiber, 4 g sugars (0 g added sugars), 13 g fat (5.5 g sat fat), 52 mg chol, 760 mg sodium

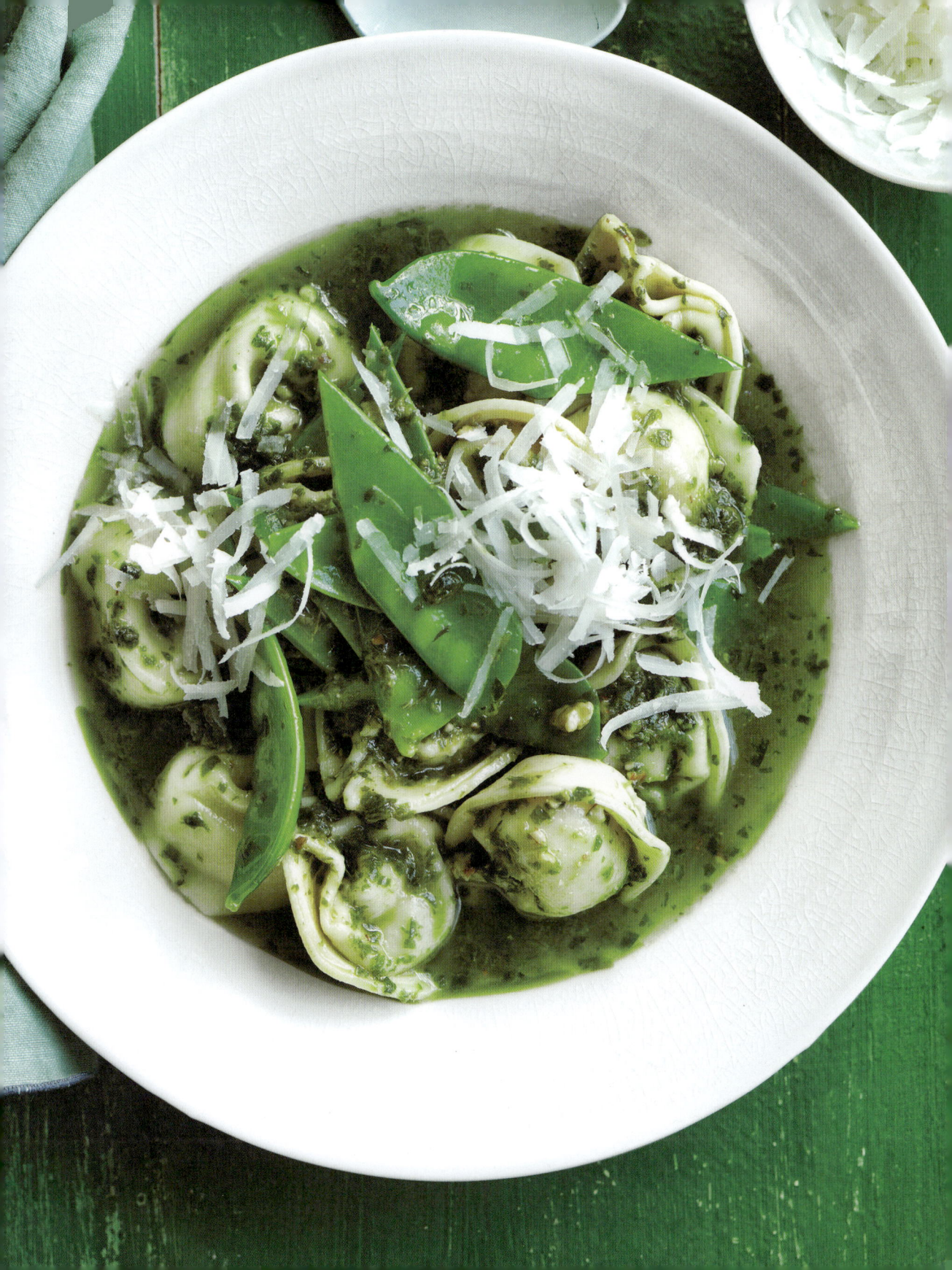

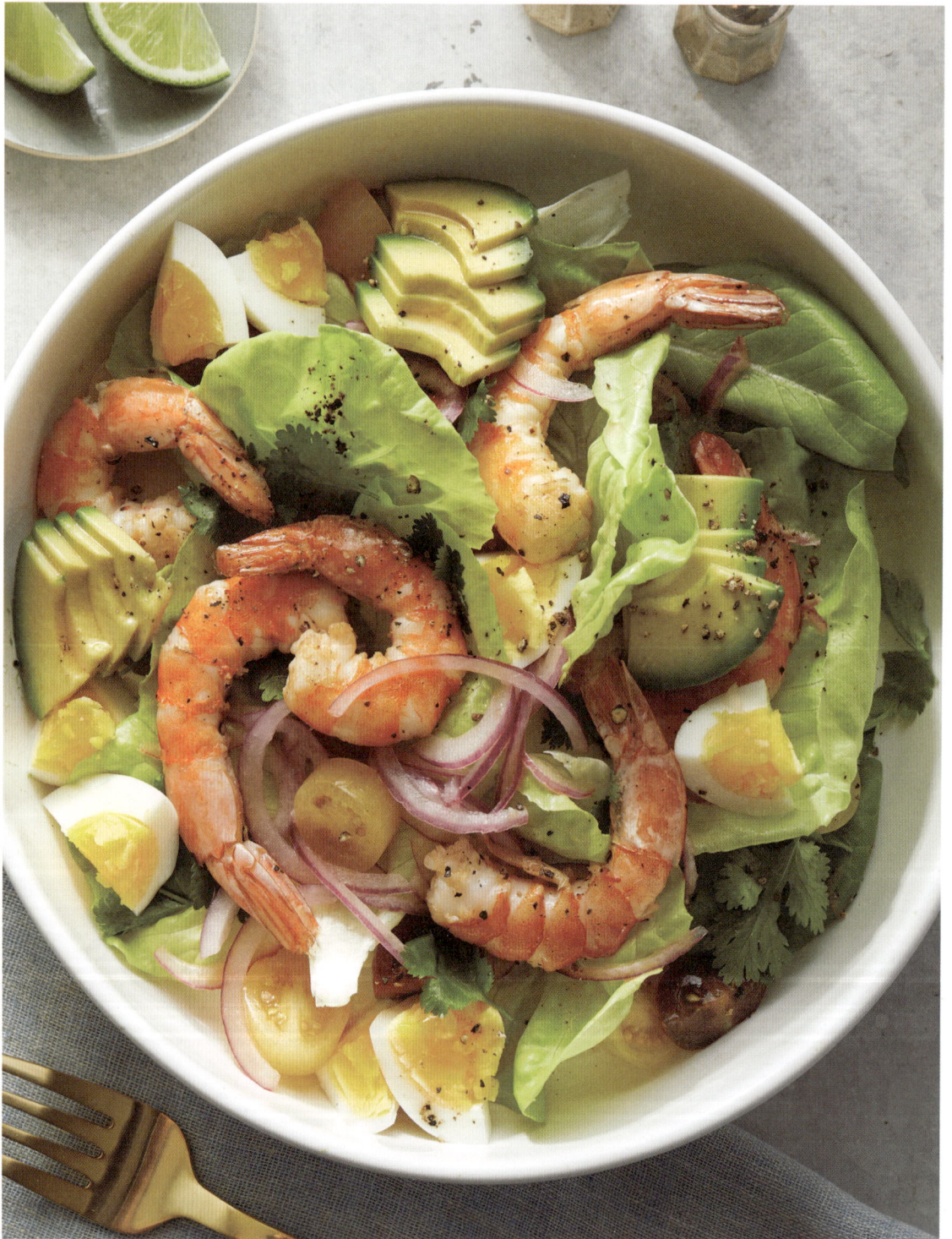

SHRIMP, AVOCADO, AND EGG CHOPPED SALAD

ACTIVE **10 MIN.**
TOTAL **15 MIN.**
SERVES **1**

⅛ small red onion, thinly sliced
1 Tbsp fresh lime juice
½ Tbsp olive oil, divided
6 oz large shrimp, peeled and deveined
   Kosher salt and pepper
½ cup grape tomatoes, halved
4 cups butter lettuce
¼ cup fresh cilantro leaves
¼ avocado, diced
1 hard boiled egg, cut into pieces

DIRECTIONS

1. In a large bowl, toss onion with lime juice and ¼ Tbsp olive oil and let sit for 5 min.

2. Heat ¼ Tbsp oil in a large skillet on medium high. Season shrimp with ⅛ tsp each salt and pepper and cook until opaque throughout, 2 to 3 min. per side.

3. Toss tomatoes with onion, then toss with lettuce and cilantro. Top with shrimp, avocado, and egg.

NUTRITION
PER SERVING 365 cal, 40 g pro, 15 g carb, 7 g fiber, 7 g sugars (0 g added sugars), 17 g fat (5 g sat fat), 450 mg chol, 600 mg sodium

WEEK 2: AT-A-GLANCE

Day 8

BREAKFAST
1 Pumpkin-Cherry Breakfast Cookie 🗆 + 2 scrambled eggs

SNACK
1 medium pear + 1 oz shelled dry-roasted pistachios (about ¼ cup) 🖊

LUNCH
Curried Tuna and Apple Salad Sandwich

SNACK
¼ cup roasted red pepper hummus + ½ seedless cucumber, sliced

DINNER
Herb-Pounded Chicken with Arugula

Day 9 - FASTING

LUNCH
Turkey Panini with Strawberry Pesto 🖊 + 1 medium pear

SNACK
¾ cup nonfat plain Greek yogurt topped with ⅓ cup blueberries, 1 Tbsp chopped walnuts, and 2 tsp honey

SNACK
Chicken Apple Quesadilla

DINNER
Tex-Mex Salmon Bowl

Day 10

BREAKFAST
2 Vegetarian Egg Muffins 🗆

SNACK
1 medium orange + 1 part-skim cheese stick

LUNCH
Curried Tuna and Apple Salad Sandwich 🍲 + Tangy Cucumber Salad

SNACK
1 Pumpkin-Cherry Breakfast Cookie 🗆

DINNER
Hot-Honey Roasted Salmon and Radishes

Day 11 - FASTING

LUNCH
Herb-Pounded Chicken with Arugula 🍲 + 1 toasted ciabatta roll

SNACK
1 Pumpkin-Cherry Breakfast Cookie 🗆 + ¾ cup nonfat plain Greek yogurt topped

SNACK
2 Vegetarian Egg Muffins 🗆

DINNER
Tex-Mex Salmon Bowl 🍲

Day 12

BREAKFAST
1 Pumpkin-Cherry Breakfast Cookies 🗆 + 2 scrambled eggs

SNACK
1 oz shelled dry-roasted pistachios (about ¼ cup) 🖊

LUNCH
Chicken Apple Quesadilla 🍲 + 1 medium orange

SNACK
¼ cup roasted red pepper hummus and ½ seedless cucumber (sliced)

DINNER
Pork Tenderloin with Roasted Red Grapes and Cabbage

Day 13 - FASTING

LUNCH
Turkey Panini with Strawberry Pesto 🍲 + ¼ cup roasted red pepper hummus and 6 baby carrots

SNACK
1 medium orange + 1 oz shelled dry-roasted pistachios (about ¼ cup)

SNACK
2 Vegetarian Egg Muffins 🗆

DINNER
Romesco Quinoa + Simple salad: Toss 1½ cup arugula or other leafy greens with 2 Tbsp vinaigrette

Day 14

BREAKFAST
Breakfast Egg Wrap

SNACK
1 medium pear with 1 Tbsp almond butter or other nut butter

LUNCH
Romesco Quinoa 🍲

SNACK
1 part-skim cheese stick + ½ cup blueberries or other berry

DINNER
Pork Tenderloin with Roasted Red Grapes and Cabbage 🍲

🗆 **Fully prepped**

🖊 **Partially prepped**

🍲 **Leftover**

SHOPPING LIST

PRODUCE

- 3   medium pears
- 1½   seedless cucumbers
- 3   green apples
- 2   lemons
- 1   celery rib
- ½   cup baby spinach
- 1½   tomato
- 12   to 14 sprigs fresh thyme
- 1   tsp fresh rosemary
- 4   cloves garlic
- 2½   cups arugula
- ¼   red onion
- ¼   small onion
- 1⅓   cups blueberries
- ½   cup basil
- 5   large strawberries
- 1   scallion
- ½   avocado
- ½   jalapeno pepper
- 1   lime
- 4   cremini mushrooms
- 3   medium oranges
- 1   bunch small red radishes (about ½ lb total)
- ¾   cup flat-leaf parsley
- ½   small purple cabbage
- 1   shallot
- ¾   cup seedless red grapes
- 6   baby carrots

MEAT & SEAFOOD

- 2   6- to 8-oz skinless, boneless chicken breasts
- 4   oz cooked, sliced turkey breasts
- 1   cup shredded rotisserie chicken breast
- 2   7-oz salmon fillets
- 2   5-oz salmon fillets
- ¾   lb pork tenderloin

REFRIGERATOR & DAIRY

- 16   eggs
- ¾   cup roasted red pepper hummus
- 1¾   cups nonfat plain Greek yogurt
- 2   Tbsp reduced-fat sour cream
- 1   Tbsp grated Parmesan
- ½   cup Gruyere
- 2   part-skim cheese sticks
- 1   oz Manchego cheese
- ¼   cup shredded Cheddar Jack cheese
- 1   oz sharp Cheddar cheese

BREAD & BAKERY

- 4   slices whole-grain bread
- 3   ciabatta rolls
- 3   tortillas

PANTRY

- 2   cups whole-wheat flour
- 1   cup old-fashioned oats
- 1   tsp baking soda
- 1   tsp pumpkin pie spice
- 1   15-oz can pure pumpkin
- 1½   cups extra-virgin olive oil
- 1   Tbsp sesame oil
- 1   cup brown sugar
- ½   cup roasted salted pepitas
- ½   cup dried cherries
- 3   oz shelled, dry-roasted pistachios
- ½   cup no-salt-added can white beans
- ¾   cup black beans
- 3   Tbsp honey
- 1   tsp curry powder
- 1   6-oz can low-sodium, water-packed chunk white tuna
- ¼   tsp red pepper flakes
- 1   tsp balsamic vinegar
- 1½   Tbsp rice vinegar
- ¼   cup red wine vinegar
- ½   Tbsp sherry vinegar
- 2   Tbsp chopped walnuts
- ¾   tsp ground cumin
- 1   cup ready-to-heat cooked brown rice
- 1   tsp reduced-sodium soy sauce
- ¾   cup chickpeas
- ⅔   cup quinoa
- 1   tsp smoked paprika
- ½   12-oz jar roasted piquillo peppers
- ½   cup almonds
- 1   Tbsp almond butter or other nut butter
- 3   squares dark chocolate

MEAL PREP DAY

Make it easy by partially prepping the day before you start your week.

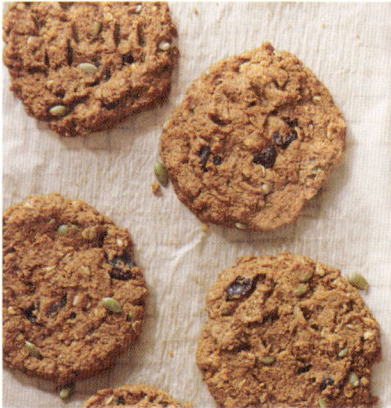

PUMPKIN-CHERRY BREAKFAST COOKIES (P. 84)

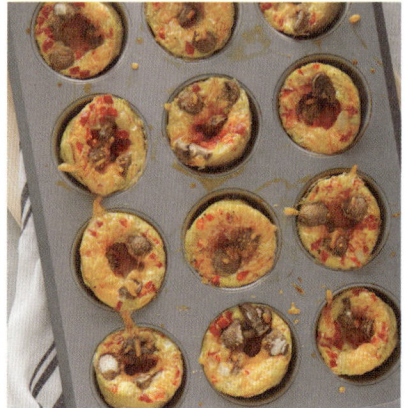

VEGETARIAN EGG MUFFINS (P. 96)

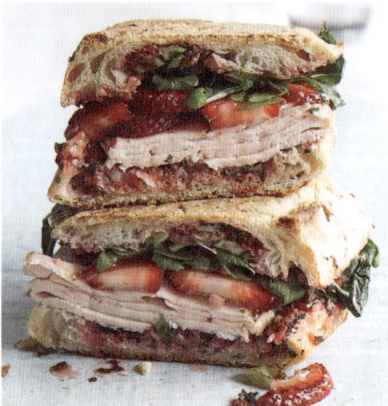

STRAWBERRY PESTO

Make strawberry pesto for Turkey Panini with Strawberry Pesto (p. 91)

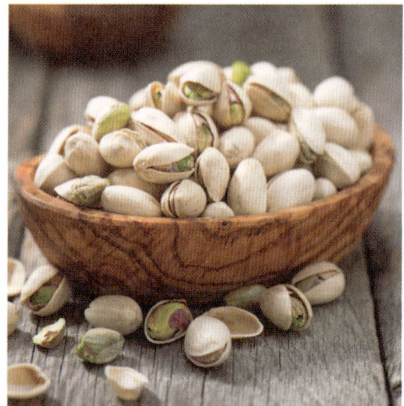

SHELLED DRY-ROASTED PISTACHIOS

Fill 3 Ziploc bags with 1 oz shelled dry-roasted pistachios each (about ¼ cup each) for snacks on Days 8, 12, and 13

MEAL PLAN
DAY 8

BREAKFAST
1 Pumpkin-Cherry
Breakfast Cookies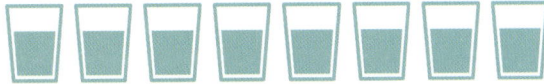
(p. 84) + 2 scrambled
eggs

SNACK
1 medium pear + 1 oz
shelled dry-roasted
pistachios (about
¼ cup)

LUNCH
Curried Tuna and Apple
Salad Sandwich (p. 87)

SNACK
¼ cup roasted red
pepper hummus +
½ seedless cucumber,
sliced

DINNER
Herb-Pounded Chicken
with Arugula (p. 88)

WATER

MOVEMENT Y ☐ N ☐

ACTIVITY	DURATION	INTENSITY

SLEEP

BEDTIME	WAKE UP

MOOD

☺ ☺ ☹

MEAL PLAN
DAY 9

LUNCH
Turkey Panini with
Strawberry Pesto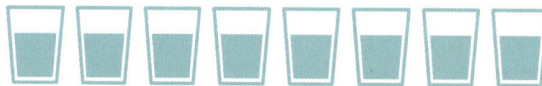
(p. 91) + 1 medium pear

SNACK
¾ cup nonfat plain
Greek yogurt topped
with ⅓ cup blueberries,
1 Tbsp chopped
walnuts, and 2 tsp
honey

SNACK
Chicken Apple
Quesadilla (p. 92)

DINNER
Tex-Mex Salmon Bowl
(p. 95)

WATER

MOVEMENT Y ☐ N ☐

ACTIVITY	DURATION	INTENSITY

SLEEP

BEDTIME	WAKE UP

MOOD

☺ ☺ ☹

MEAL PLAN
DAY 10

BREAKFAST
2 Vegetarian Egg
Muffins 🍽 (p. 96)

SNACK
1 medium orange +
1 part-skim cheese stick

LUNCH
Curried Tuna and
Apple Salad Sandwich
🍽 + Tangy Cucumber
Salad: Toss ½ seedless
cucumber (sliced) with
1½ Tbsp rice vinegar,
1 Tbsp sesame oil and
1 tsp reduced-sodium
soy sauce. Let stand
5 min.

SNACK
1 Pumpkin-Cherry
Breakfast Cookies 🍽

DINNER
Hot-Honey Roasted
Salmon and Radishes
(p. 99)

WATER

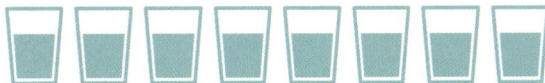

MOVEMENT Y☐ N☐

ACTIVITY	DURATION	INTENSITY

SLEEP

BEDTIME	WAKE UP

MOOD

☺ ☻ ☹

MEAL PLAN
DAY 11

↓

FASTING DAY

LUNCH
Herb-Pounded Chicken with Arugula 🍲 +
1 toasted ciabatta roll

SNACK
1 Pumpkin-Cherry Breakfast Cookies 🍪
+ ¾ cup nonfat plain Greek yogurt topped with ⅓ cup blueberries, 1 Tbsp chopped walnuts, and 2 tsp honey

SNACK
2 Vegetarian Egg Muffins 🍪

DINNER
Tex-Mex Salmon Bowl 🍲

WATER

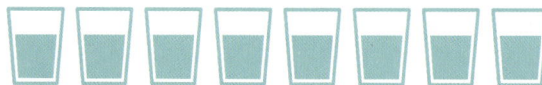

MOVEMENT Y ☐ N ☐

ACTIVITY	DURATION	INTENSITY

SLEEP

BEDTIME	WAKE UP

MOOD

🙂 😐 🙁

MEAL PLAN
DAY 12

BREAKFAST
1 Pumpkin-Cherry
Breakfast Cookies
+ 2 scrambled eggs

SNACK
1 oz shelled dry-roasted
pistachios (about
¼ cup)

LUNCH
Chicken Apple
Quesadilla +
1 medium orange

SNACK
¼ cup roasted red
pepper hummus and
½ seedless cucumber
(sliced)

DINNER
Pork Tenderloin with
Roasted Red Grapes and
Cabbage (p. 100)

WATER

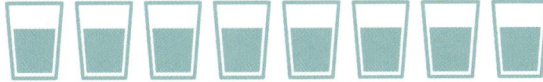

MOVEMENT Y ☐ N ☐

ACTIVITY	DURATION	INTENSITY

SLEEP

BEDTIME	WAKE UP

MOOD

☺ ☺ ☹

MEAL PLAN
DAY 13

↓
FASTING DAY

LUNCH
Turkey Panini with Strawberry Pesto 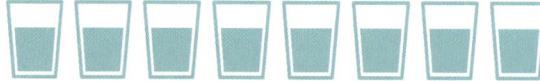 +
¼ cup roasted red pepper hummus and 6 baby carrots

SNACK
1 medium orange +
1 oz shelled dry-roasted pistachios (about ¼ cup)

SNACK
2 Vegetarian Egg Muffins

DINNER
Romesco Quinoa (p. 103) + Simple salad: Toss 1½ cup arugula or other leafy greens with 2 Tbsp vinaigrette.

WATER

MOVEMENT   Y ☐ N ☐

ACTIVITY	DURATION	INTENSITY

SLEEP

BEDTIME	WAKE UP

MOOD

:) :| :(

MEAL PLAN
DAY 14

BREAKFAST
Breakfast Egg Wrap:
Place 2 scrambled eggs
in the center of a flour
tortilla. Top with ¼ cup
shredded Cheddar Jack
or other cheese. Serve
with salsa, if desired.

SNACK
1 medium pear with
1 Tbsp almond butter or
other nut butter

LUNCH
Romesco Quinoa

SNACK
1 part-skim cheese stick
+ ½ cup blueberries or
other berry

DINNER
Pork Tenderloin with
Roasted Red Grapes and
Cabbage

WATER

MOVEMENT Y ☐ N ☐

ACTIVITY	DURATION	INTENSITY

SLEEP

BEDTIME	WAKE UP

MOOD

☺ ☺ ☹

PUMPKIN-CHERRY BREAKFAST COOKIES

ACTIVE **15 MIN.**
TOTAL **1 HR.**
MAKES **16**

2	cups whole-wheat flour
1	cup old-fashioned oats
1	tsp baking soda
1	tsp pumpkin pie spice
½	tsp kosher salt
1	15-oz can pure pumpkin
1	cup olive oil
1	cup brown sugar
1	large egg
½	cup roasted salted pepitas
½	cup dried cherries

DIRECTIONS

1. Heat oven to 350°F. In a medium bowl, whisk together flour, oats, baking soda, pie spice, and salt.

2. Using an electric mixer, beat pumpkin, oil, sugar, and egg on medium to combine. Reduce speed to low; gradually incorporate flour mixture, then pepitas and cherries.

3. Scoop 16 mounds (about ⅓ cup each) onto parchment-lined baking sheets, spacing 2 in. apart; flatten into disks. Bake until dark brown on bottoms, 20 to 25 min. Transfer to wire rack to cool.

NUTRITION
PER COOKIE 290 cal, 4 g pro, 33 g carb, 3 g fiber, 16 g sugars (13.5 g added sugars), 16.5 g fat (2.5 g sat fat), 11.5 mg chol, 160 mg sodium

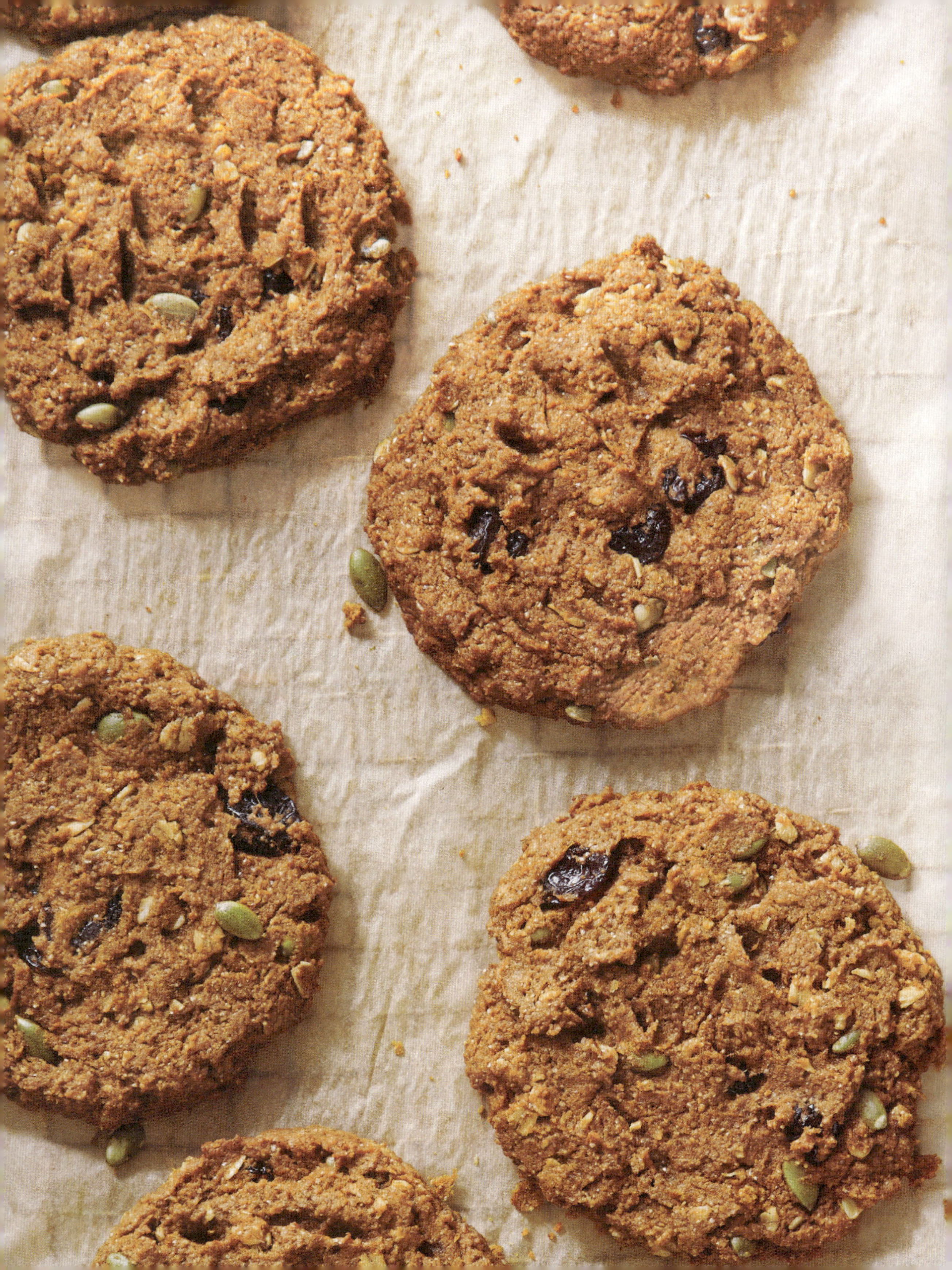

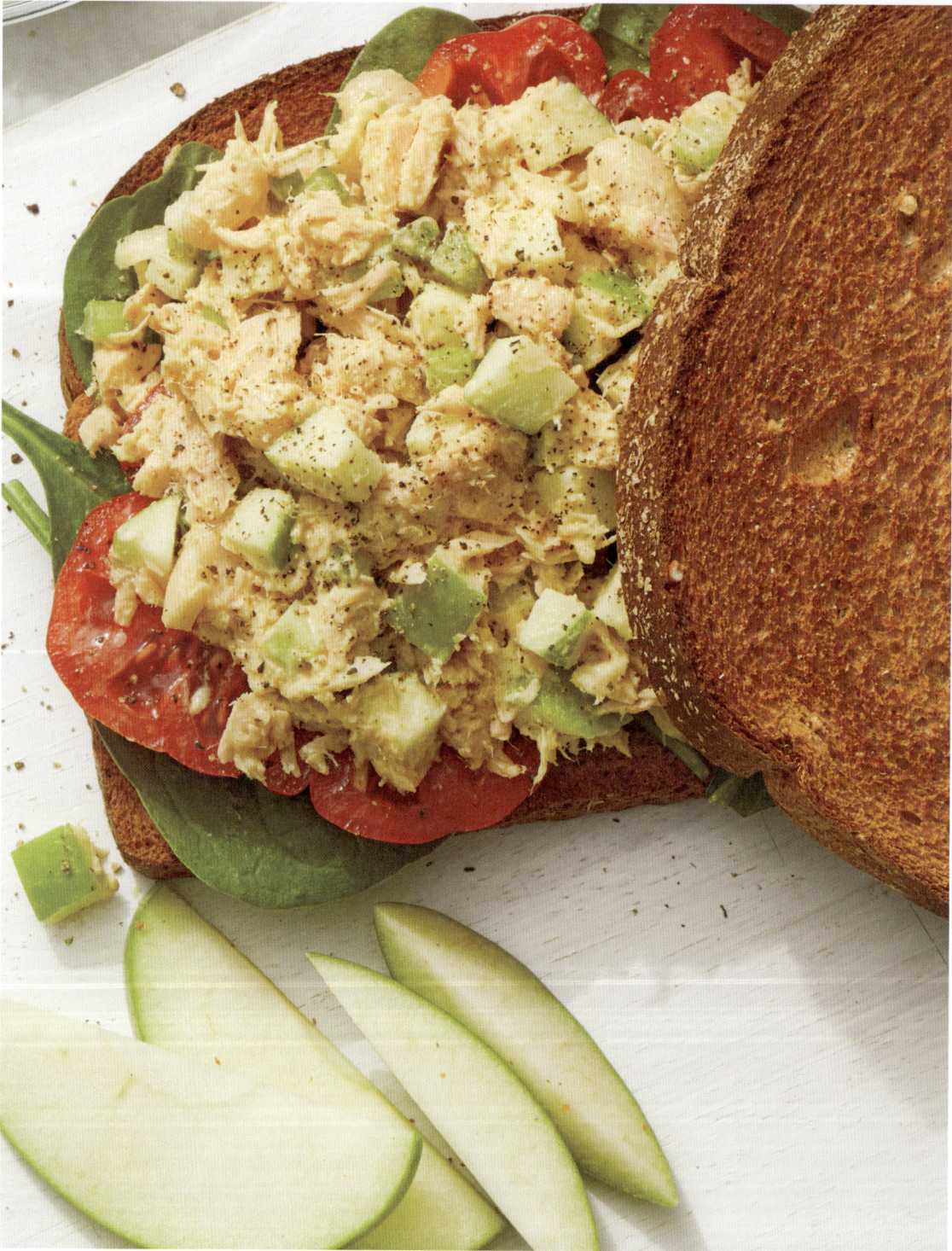

CURRIED TUNA AND APPLE SALAD SANDWICH

ACTIVE **20 MIN.**
TOTAL **20 MIN.**
SERVES **2**

2	tart green apples, halved
½	cup no-salt-added canned white beans, rinsed and drained
3	Tbsp nonfat plain Greek yogurt
2	Tbsp reduced-fat sour cream
2	tsp fresh lemon juice
1	tsp honey
1	tsp curry powder
1	can (6-oz) low-sodium water-packed chunk white tuna, drained
1	rib celery, chopped
½	cup baby spinach
1	tomato, thinly sliced
4	slices whole-grain bread, thinly sliced

DIRECTIONS

1. Chop ½ apple and set aside for the salad. Cut the remaining 1½ apples into wedges for serving.

2. In a medium bowl, mash the beans with the back of a spoon or a potato masher. Add the yogurt, sour cream, lemon juice, honey, and curry powder. Stir until combined.

3. Add the tuna, celery, and chopped apple. Stir until combined. Arrange the spinach and tomato on 2 slices of bread. Top with the tuna and remaining bread slices. Cut the sandwiches in half and serve with the apple wedges.

NUTRITION
PER SERVING 430 cal, 37 g pro, 60 g carb, 11 g fiber, 24 g sugars (7 g added sugars), 7 g fat (2 g sat fat), 45 mg chol, 310 mg sodium

HERB-POUNDED CHICKEN WITH ARUGULA

ACTIVE **5 MIN.**
TOTAL **30 MIN.**
SERVES **2**

2	6- to 8-oz boneless, skinless chicken breasts
3	Tbsp extra-virgin olive oil, divided
1	small lemon, zested plus wedges for serving
2	tsp chopped fresh thyme
1	tsp chopped fresh rosemary
1	small clove garlic, chopped
¼	tsp red pepper flakes
	Kosher salt
2	cups arugula
¼	red onion, thinly sliced
1	tsp balsamic vinegar

DIRECTIONS

1. Starting at the thicker side, make a lengthwise cut into the side of the chicken breasts about two-thirds of the way in. Fold the breasts open like a book.

2. In a bowl, mix 1 Tbsp oil, lemon zest, thyme, rosemary, garlic, red pepper, and a big pinch of salt. Rub this mixture all over the chicken. Place each chicken breast between two pieces of plastic wrap and using a meat mallet (or bottom of a heavy pan), pound the breasts to a ¼-in. thickness.

3. In a large skillet over medium-high, heat 1 Tbsp olive oil. Add a chicken breast and sear on both sides, about 3 min. each. Transfer to a plate and repeat with the other breast.

4. In a medium bowl, toss the arugula, onion, balsamic, and the remaining Tbsp olive oil. Squeeze a wedge of lemon over the chicken and serve with the arugula salad.

NUTRITION
PER SERVING 330 cal, 26 g pro, 3 g carb, 1 g fiber, 1 g sugars (0 g added sugars), 23.5 g fat (3.5 g sat fat), 85 mg chol, 300 mg sodium

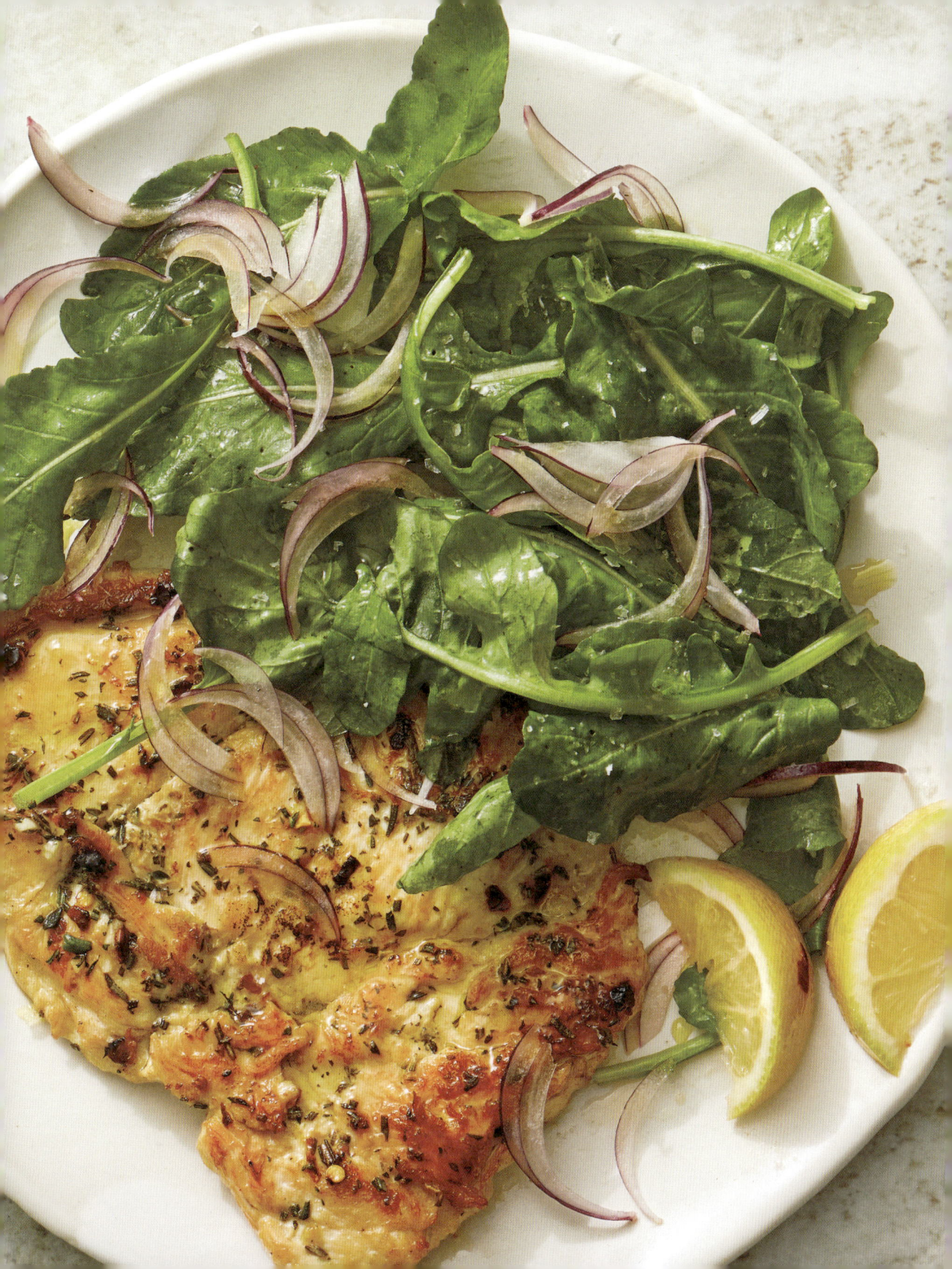

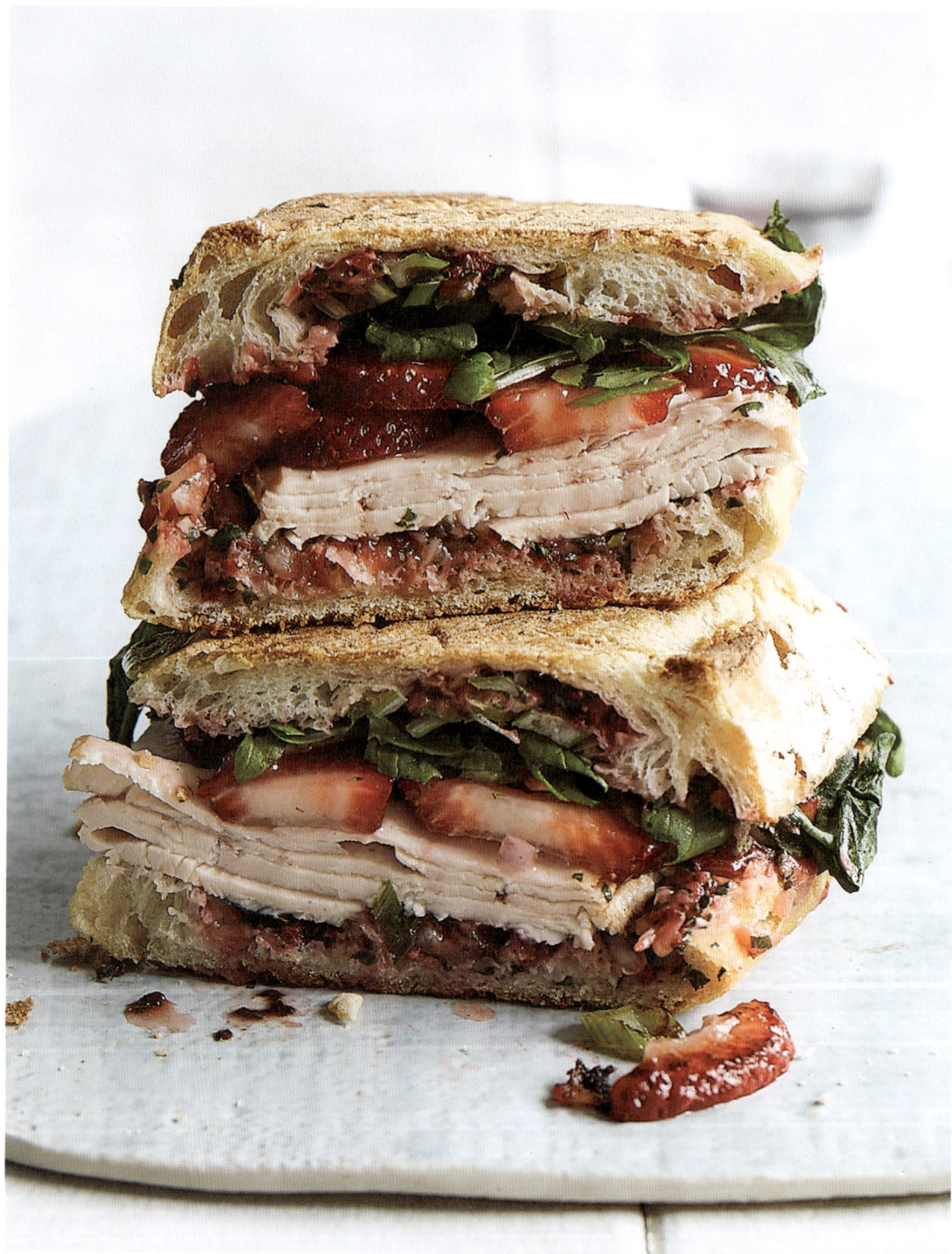

TURKEY PANINI WITH STRAWBERRY PESTO

ACTIVE **40 MIN.**
TOTAL **50 MIN.**
SERVES **2**

½	cup basil leaves
1	Tbsp grated Parmesan
1	Tbsp olive oil
½	Tbsp lemon juice
½	clove garlic
5	large strawberries, hulled
2	ciabatta rolls, halved
4	oz cooked turkey breast, sliced
½	cup baby arugula
1	scallion, chopped

DIRECTIONS

1. In a mini food processor, blend basil, Parmesan, oil, lemon juice, and garlic until smooth. Add half the strawberries and pulse until finely chopped.

2. Slice remaining strawberries. Spread pesto on both halves of each roll. Divide turkey, arugula, sliced berries, and scallions among halves; sandwich with remaining halves.

3. Heat a large skillet on medium-high. Place panini in skillet and press with a second skillet. Cook until golden brown, 2 to 3 min. per side. Repeat with remaining panini. Cut each sandwich in half before serving.

NUTRITION

PER SERVING 360 cal, 26 g pro, 42 g carb, 3 g fiber, 3 g sugars (1 g added sugar), 9.5 g fat (1.5 g sat fat), 49 mg chol, 590 mg sodium

CHICKEN APPLE QUESADILLA

ACTIVE **10 MIN.**
TOTAL **10 MIN.**
SERVES **1**

1	**tortilla**
¼	**cup shredded Gruyere**
½	**cup shredded cooked chicken breast**
6	**thin apple slices**
	Salsa, for serving

DIRECTIONS

1. In a large skillet on medium heat, heat the tortilla.

2. Mix shredded Gruyere and shredded cooked chicken breast and spread over half the tortilla.

3. Layer apple slices on top of chicken mixture and fold tortilla over like an omelet. Cook, flipping once, until edges brown and cheese melts, about 5 min. Cut into wedges. Serve with salsa if desired.

NUTRITION

PER SERVING 330 cal, 33 g pro, 31 g carb, 2 g fiber, 5 g sugars (0 g added sugars), 14 g fat (6 g sat fat), 90 mg chol, 640 mg sodium

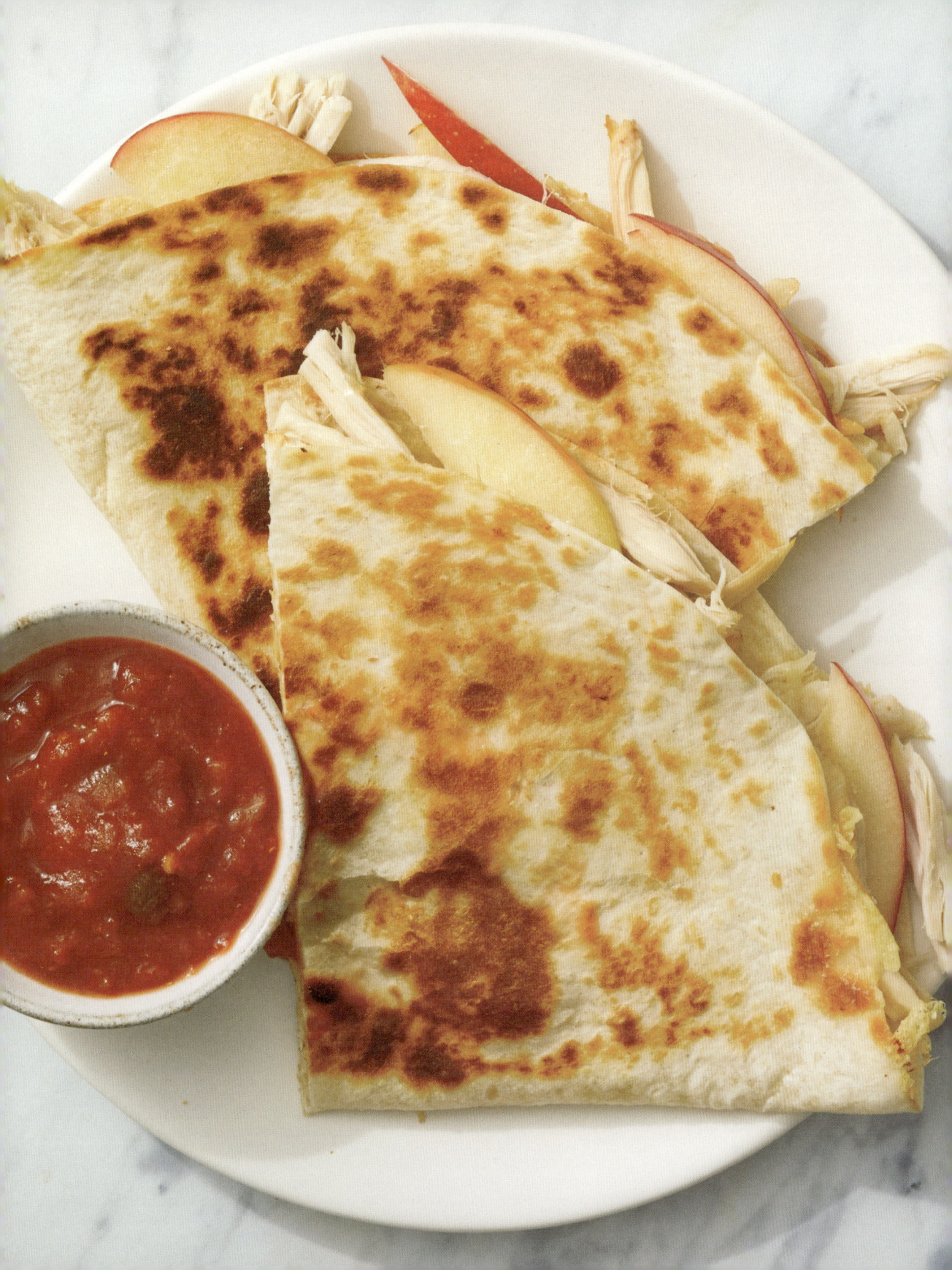

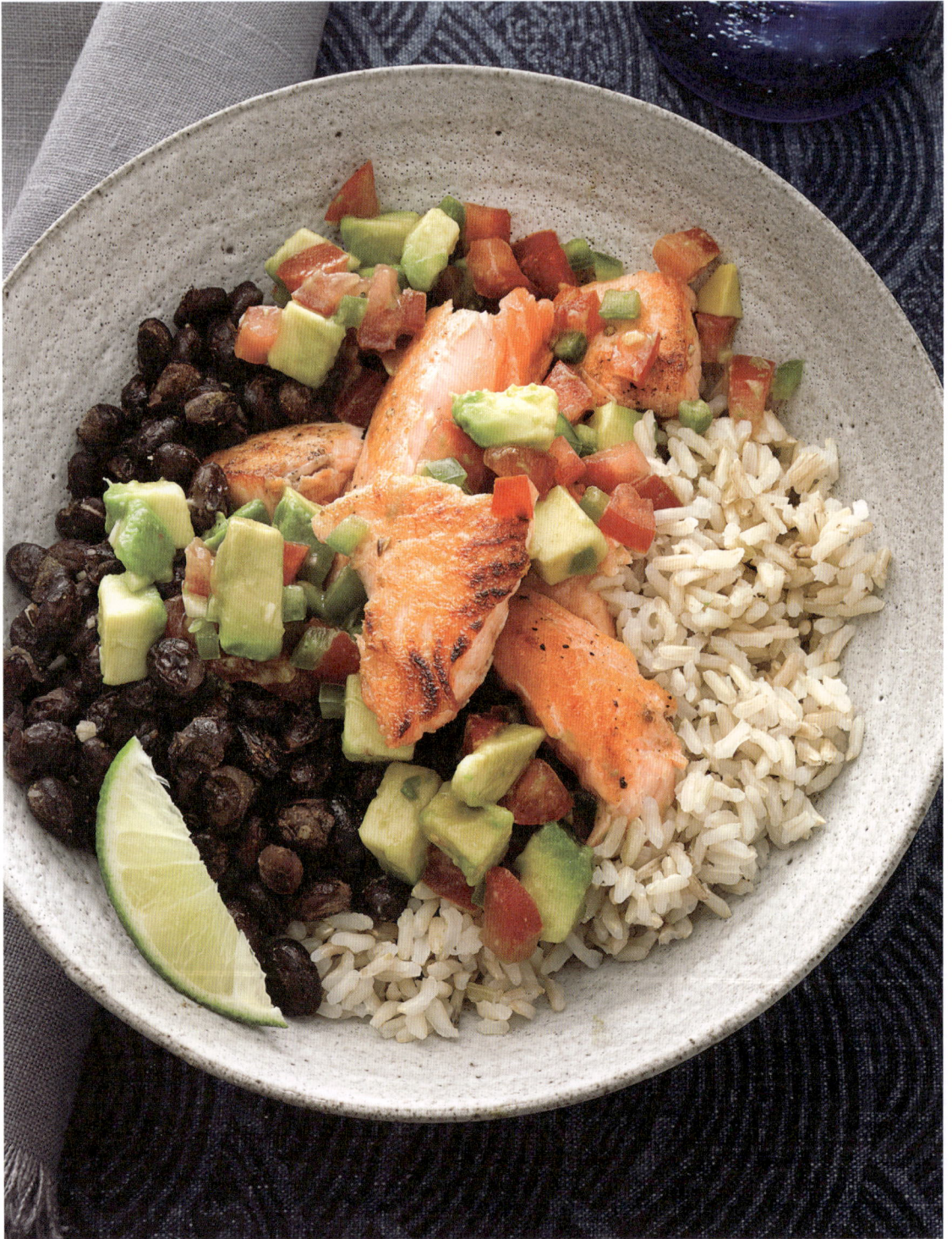

TEX-MEX SALMON BOWL

ACTIVE **15 MIN.**
TOTAL **20 MIN.**
SERVES **2**

½ avocado, cut into pieces
½ medium tomato, cut into ¼-in. pieces
¼ jalapeño, seeded and finely chopped
1½ Tbsp fresh lime juice, divided
Kosher salt and pepper
2 7-oz skinless salmon fillets
1½ cloves garlic, finely chopped, divided
½ Tbsp plus ½ tsp olive oil, divided
¾ tsp ground cumin, divided
¾ cup black beans, rinsed
1 cup cooked brown rice

DIRECTIONS

1. Toss avocado, tomato, and jalapeño with ½ Tbsp lime juice and ¼ tsp salt. Refrigerate, covered, until ready to use.

2. In a bowl, toss salmon with ½ Tbsp lime juice, two-thirds of garlic, ½ tsp oil, ½ tsp cumin, and ¼ tsp salt. Heat remaining ½ Tbsp oil in a large nonstick skillet on medium. Add salmon and cook until nearly opaque throughout, 3 to 4 min. per side; transfer to plates.

3. Discard half of oil from skillet, add remaining garlic and cook on medium, stirring, 1 minute. Add beans and remaining ½ Tbsp lime juice and ¼ tsp cumin and cook, stirring, until heated through, about 2 min.

4. Flake salmon and serve with rice, beans, and avocado salsa.

NUTRITION
PER SERVING 600 cal, 53 g pro, 47 g carb, 12 g fiber, 2.5 g sugars (0 g added sugars), 23 g fat (4 g sat fat), 89 mg chol, 690 mg sodium

VEGETARIAN EGG MUFFINS

ACTIVE **5 MIN.**
TOTAL **25 MIN.**
MAKES **6**

5   **large eggs plus 4 egg whites**
    Kosher salt and pepper
½   **red pepper**
4   **small cremini mushrooms, quartered**
¼   **small onion, finely chopped**
1   **oz sharp Cheddar cheese, coarsely grated (about ¼ cup)**

DIRECTIONS

1. Heat oven to 350°F and spray a 6-cup muffin pan with cooking spray.

2. In a large bowl, whisk together eggs, egg whites, and ⅛ tsp each salt and pepper. Stir in red pepper, mushrooms, onion, and Cheddar.

3. Divide the mixture among the cups and bake until just set, 10 to 20 min.

NUTRITION

PER SERVING (2 MUFFINS) 220 cal, 18 g pro, 5 g carb, 4 g fiber, 2 g sugars (0 g added sugars), 11 g fat, 4 g sat fat, 318 mg chol, 300 mg sodium

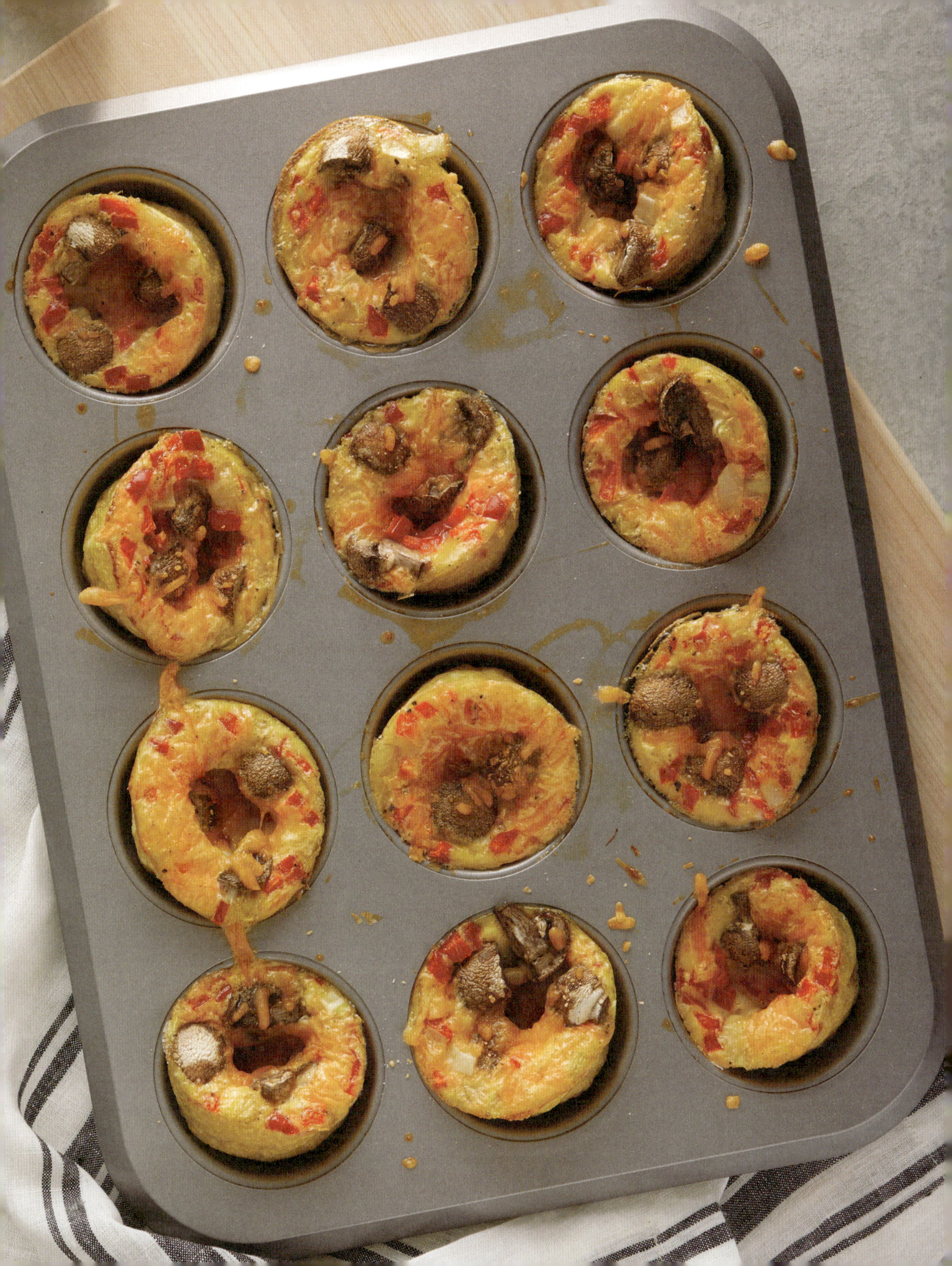

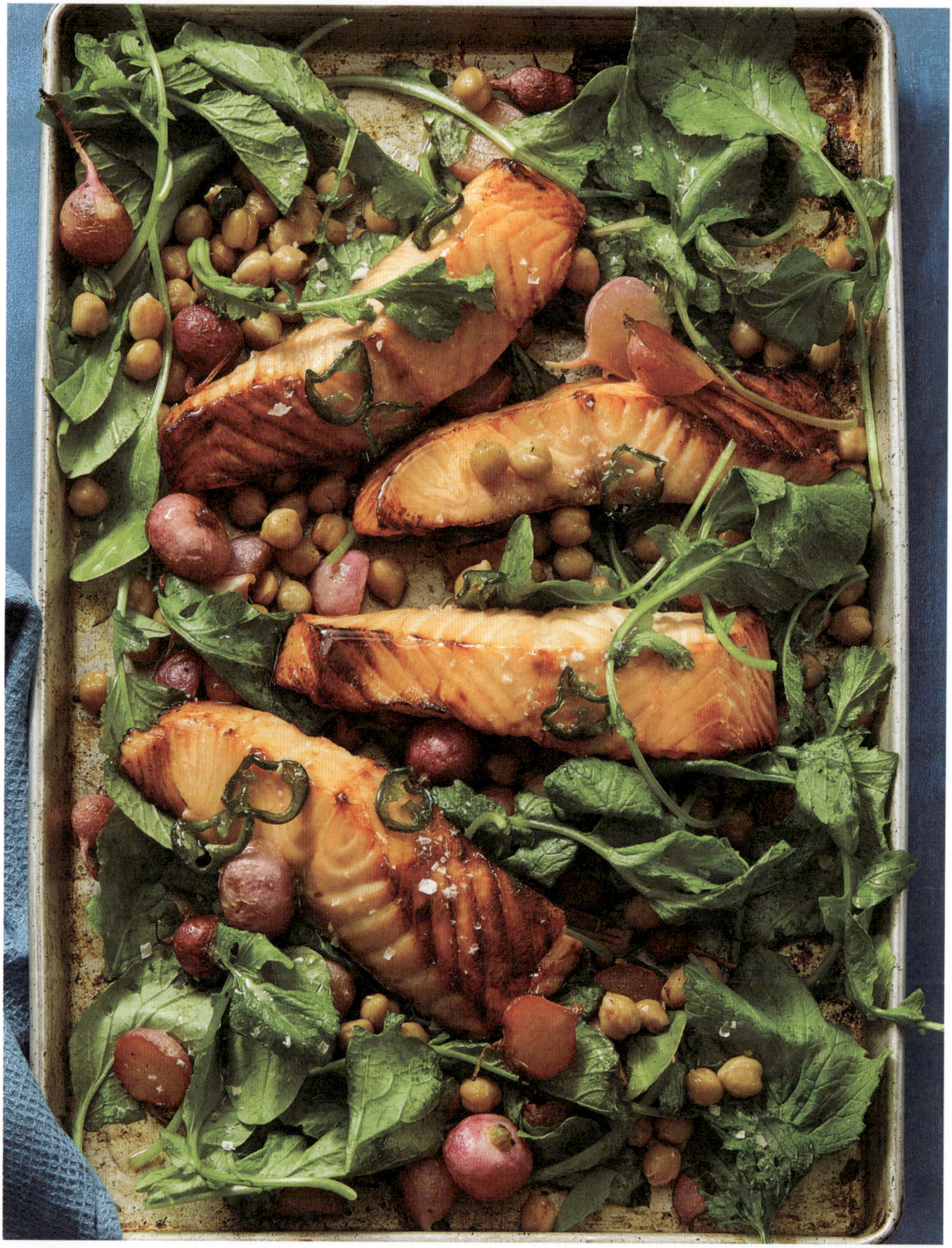

HOT-HONEY ROASTED SALMON AND RADISHES

ACTIVE **15 MIN.**
TOTAL **35 MIN.**
SERVES **2**

1   Tbsp honey
¼   jalapeño, thinly sliced
1   bunch small red radishes (about ½ lb total), halved (or quartered if very large), greens reserved
½   Tbsp olive oil
      Kosher salt and pepper
2   5-oz salmon fillets
¾   cup chickpeas, rinsed

DIRECTIONS

1. Heat oven to 425°F. In a small saucepan, bring honey and jalapeño to a simmer. Remove from heat and let sit 5 min., then remove and set aside jalapeño slices for serving.

2. On a large rimmed baking sheet, toss radishes with oil and ¼ tsp each salt and pepper; push to edges of sheet.

3. Place salmon in center of sheet, drizzle with 1½ Tbsp honey mixture, and season with ¼ tsp each salt and pepper. Roast until radishes are tender and salmon is opaque throughout, 15 to 20 min.

4. Transfer salmon to plates and drizzle with remaining ½ Tbsp honey mixture. Toss radishes with chickpeas, then radish greens. Serve with salmon.

NUTRITION

PER SERVING 250 cal, 34 g pro, 29 g carb, 6 g fiber, 13 g sugars (8.5 g added sugars), 10.5 g fat (2 g sat fat), 66 mg chol, 480 mg sodium

PORK TENDERLOIN WITH ROASTED RED GRAPES AND CABBAGE

ACTIVE **20 MIN.**
TOTAL **25 MIN.**
SERVES **2**

3	Tbsp olive oil, divided
2	sprigs thyme, broken into pieces
½	small purple cabbage (about ¼ lb), cut into ½-in. wedges
1	shallot, halved
¾	cup small red seedless grapes
	Kosher salt and pepper
¾	lb pork tenderloin, cut into 4 portions
¼	cup red wine vinegar

DIRECTIONS

1. Heat oven to 450°F. Evenly coat rimmed baking sheet with 2 Tbsp oil. Scatter thyme sprigs over sheet, then place cabbage in single layer on top. In open spaces, place shallots cut sides down. Scatter grapes over top and season everything with ¼ tsp each salt and pepper. Roast until cabbage is tender, shallots are caramelized, and grapes are beginning to break down and release some juices, 15 to 18 min.

2. Meanwhile, heat remaining Tbsp oil in a medium skillet on medium. Season pork with ¼ tsp each salt and pepper and cook, turning occasionally, until golden brown on all sides and instant-read thermometer inserted in center registers 145°F, 8 to 10 min. total. Transfer to cutting board and let rest at least 5 min. before slicing.

3. Remove baking sheet from oven and immediately pour vinegar onto sheet, stirring to loosen any browned bits. Slice pork and serve with cabbage, shallots, and grapes. Tip sheet to the side to collect sauce and spoon over pork and vegetables.

NUTRITION
PER SERVING 380 cal, 37 g pro, 23 g carb, 4 g fiber, 15 g sugars (0 g added sugars), 15.5 g fat (3 g sat fat), 95 mg chol, 595 mg sodium

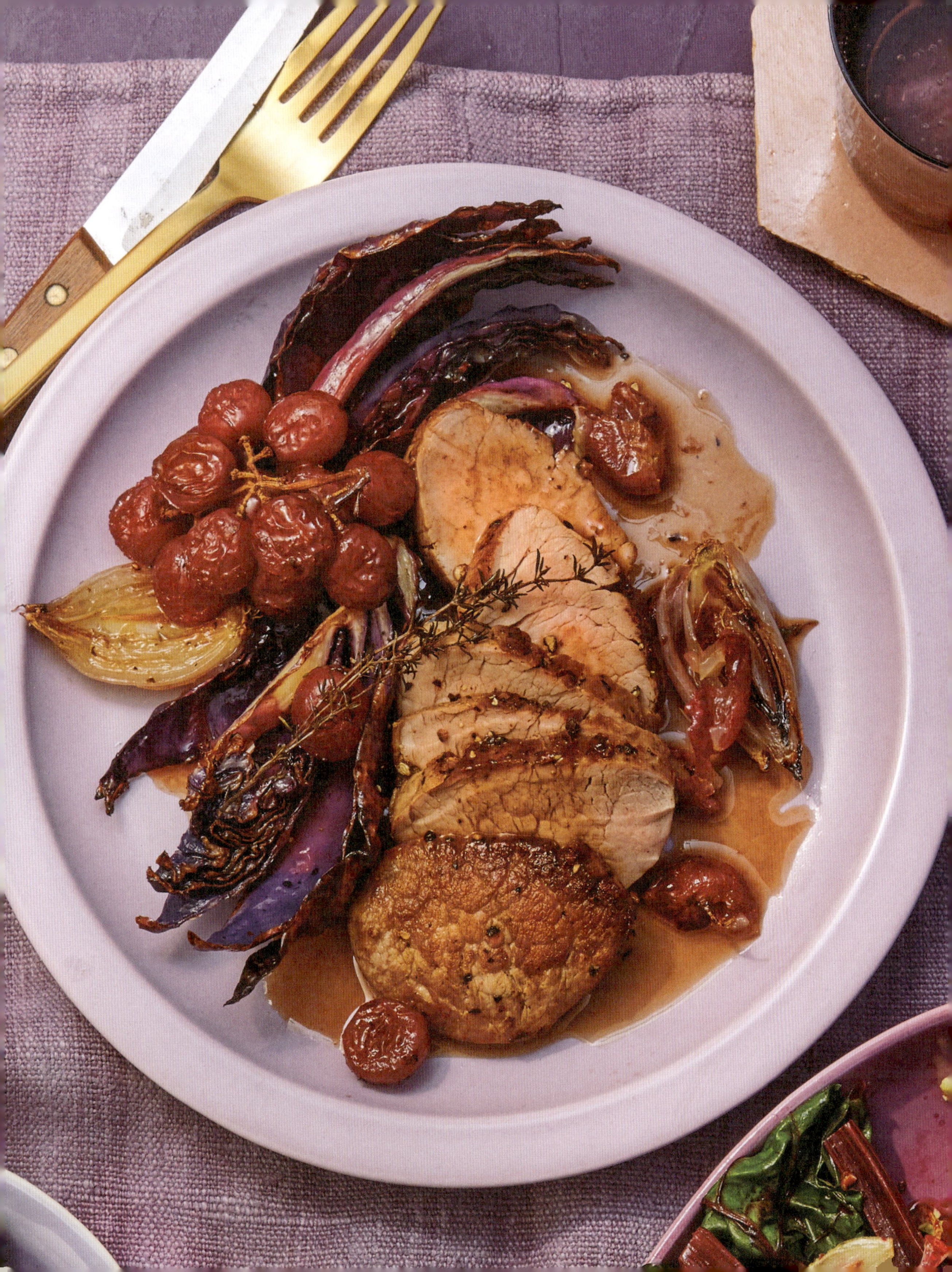

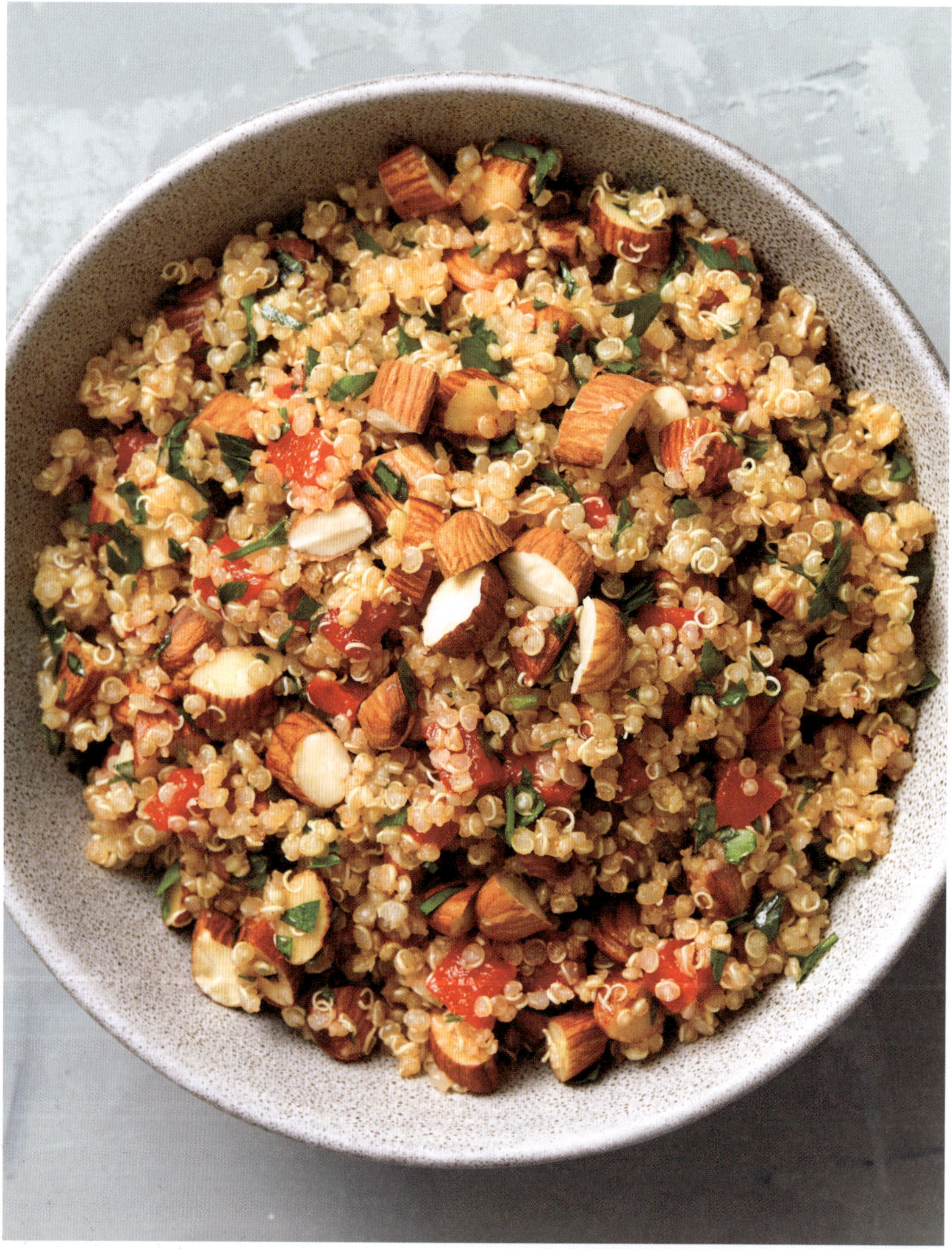

ROMESCO QUINOA

ACTIVE **15 MIN.**
TOTAL **25 MIN.**
SERVES **2**

1   ⅔ cups quinoa
1   Tbsp olive oil
½   Tbsp sherry vinegar
½   tsp grated garlic
    Kosher salt
1   tsp smoked paprika
½   12-oz jar roasted piquillo peppers, drained and chopped
½   cup almonds, well toasted and chopped, plus more for serving
¾   cup flat-leaf parsley, chopped
1   oz Manchego cheese, grated, plus more for serving

DIRECTIONS

1. In a medium saucepan, combine quinoa and 1¼ cups water and simmer until just tender, about 12 min. Remove from heat and keep covered 3 min., then fluff with a fork.

2. In a large bowl, whisk together olive oil, sherry vinegar, garlic, ½ tsp salt, and paprika. Fluff quinoa, then add to dressing and toss to combine. Add piquillo peppers, almonds, parsley and Manchego and toss well. Top with additional almonds and cheese if desired.

NUTRITION
PER SERVING 565 cal, 19 g pro, 50 g carb, 9 g fiber, 5.5 g sugars (0 g added sugars), 33 g fat (6 g sat fat), 15 mg chol, 665 mg sodium

WEEK 3: AT-A-GLANCE

Day 15

BREAKFAST
Easiest-Ever Bagels 🗀

SNACK
1 cup cubed honeydew or other melon, ½ oz walnuts (about 7 to 8 halves), and 1 part-skim cheese stick

LUNCH
Crunchy Turkey Salad

SNACK
2 Almond and Maple Energy Bites 🗀

DINNER
Pork, Pineapple, and Red Onion Kebabs + ½ cup cooked brown rice 🔪

Day 16 - FASTING

LUNCH
Caprese Chicken Pasta 🔪 + ⅔ cup pineapple cubes

SNACK
Apple-Cinnamon Yogurt

SNACK
Easiest-Ever Bagels 🍲 with 2 Tbsp creamy peanut butter

DINNER
Wild Salmon Salad

Day 17

BREAKFAST
Cheesy Avocado Omelet

SNACK
Berry Protein Smoothie

LUNCH
Crunchy Turkey Salad 🍲 + 1 cup cubed honeydew or other melon

SNACK
2 Almond Maple Energy Bites 🍲

DINNER
Seared Coconut-Lime Chicken with Snap Pea Slaw + ½ cup cooked brown rice 🔪

Day 18 - FASTING

LUNCH
Wild Salmon Salad 🍲 + ⅔ cup pineapple cubes

SNACK
Cheesy Bagel 🔪

SNACK
1 cup cubed honeydew or other melon, ½ oz walnuts (about 7 to 8 halves), and 1 part-skim cheese stick

DINNER
Peanut Sauce Soba with Crispy Tofu

Day 19

BREAKFAST
Avocado Everything Bagel 🔪

SNACK
1 cup cubed honeydew or other melon + 1 part-skim cheese stick

LUNCH
Pork, Pineapple, and Red Onion Kebabs 🍲 + ½ cup cooked brown rice 🔪

SNACK
Apple-Cinnamon Yogurt

DINNER
Baked Halibut with Potatoes and Brussels Sprouts

Day 20 - FASTING

LUNCH
Peanut Sauce Soba with Crispy Tofu 🍲

SNACK
Berry Protein Smoothie

SNACK
1 part-skim cheese stick

DINNER
Caprese Chicken Pasta 🍲 + Simple salad

Day 21

BREAKFAST
Oatmeal with Greens, Tomato, and Egg

SNACK
1 cup cubed honeydew or other melon, ½ oz walnuts (about 7 to 8 halves), and 1 part-skim cheese stick

LUNCH
Seared Coconut-Lime Chicken with Snap Pea Slaw 🍲 + ½ cup cooked brown rice 🔪

SNACK
Berry Protein Smoothie

DINNER
Baked Halibut with Potatoes and Brussels Sprouts 🍲

🗀 **Fully prepped**

🔪 **Partially prepped**

🍲 **Leftover**

104

SHOPPING LIST

PRODUCE

- 5 cups honeydew
- 2½ Tbsp fresh lime juice
- ½ Napa cabbage
- ⅛ red cabbage
- 5 scallions
- 1 Cara Cara orange
- 1 medium carrot
- 1 medium red onion
- 2⅓ cups pineapple
- 3¾ cups cherry or grape tomatoes
- ⅓ cup fresh basil
- 2 small apples
- 2.5 oz mixed baby greens
- 1¼ avocado
- 3 cremini mushrooms
- 5¾ cups baby spinach
- 2 Tbsp flat-leaf parsley
- ½ Tbsp plus ⅛ tsp grated fresh ginger
- 5 oz snap peas
- 2 oz snow peas
- ¼ cup cilantro
- 1 tsp grated garlic
- 1 Tbsp mixed fresh herbs (such as parsley, thyme, and rosemary)
- ½ lb fingerling potatoes
- ½ lb Brussels sprouts
- ½ shallot

MEAT & SEAFOOD

- 2½ cups shredded rotisserie or cooked chicken
- ¾ lb pork loin
- 2 4-oz skinless wild salmon fillets
- 1 8-oz boneless, skinless chicken breasts
- ¾ lb halibut fillet

REFRIGERATOR & DAIRY

- 2 cups plain Greek yogurt
- 2½ cups fat-free plain yogurt
- 5 eggs
- 4 part-skim cheese stick
- 2 oz fresh mozzarella pearls
- 1 oz sharp Cheddar cheese
- 3 cups unsweetened almond milk
- ½ cup shredded part-skim mozzarella cheese
- 1 12.3-oz package extra-firm tofu

FROZEN

- 3 cups frozen mixed berries

PANTRY

- 2 cups self-rising flour
- 2 tsp sesame seeds
- 2 tsp poppy seeds
- 2 tsp onion flakes
- 2½ tsp Everything Bagel seasoning
- 1½ oz whole walnuts
- 4 Tbsp chopped walnuts
- 3 Tbsp toasted sesame oil
- 1 Tbsp rice vinegar
- 3 Tbsp balsamic vinegar
- 2 tsp brown sugar
- ¼ tsp red pepper flakes
- ¼ cup crunchy chow mein noodles
- 4 oz soba noodles
- ¼ cup roasted almonds
- ¼ cup slivered almonds
- ¼ cup almond butter
- 2 Tbsp maple syrup
- ½ Tbsp chia seeds
- ¼ tsp pure vanilla extract
- ½ cup old-fashioned oats
- ¼ cup quick-cooking steel-cut oats
- ¼ cup bittersweet chocolate chips
- ½ tsp chili powder
- ¼ tsp ground cumin
- 6 Tbsp olive oil
- 2 cups brown rice
- 4 oz whole-grain penne
- 1 Tbsp honey
- ½ tsp ground cinnamon
- 3½ Tbsp natural creamy peanut butter
- 3 scoops protein powder
- 1 Tbsp coconut cream
- 1½ Tbsp canola oil
- 1¼ Tbsp reduced-sodium soy sauce
- ½ tsp sriracha
- ⅓ cup cornstarch
- 4 squares dark chocolate

MEAL PREP DAY

Make it easy by partially prepping the day before you start your week.

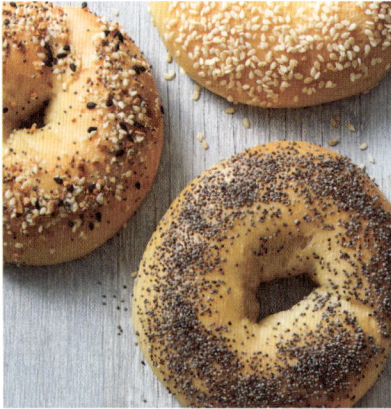

EASIEST-EVER BAGELS (P. 114)

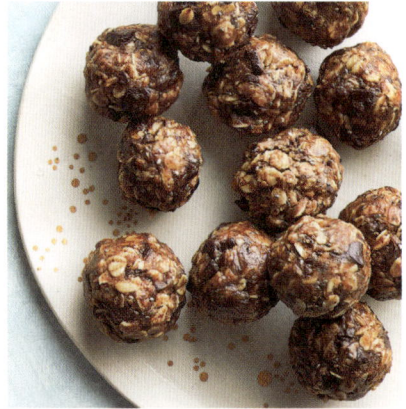

**ALMOND AND MAPLE
ENERGY BITES (P. 118)**

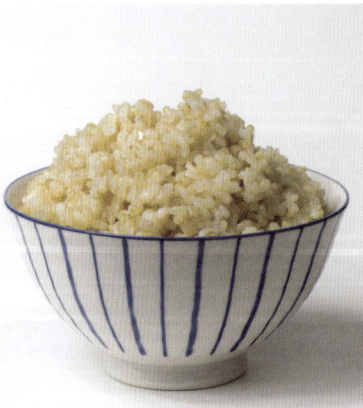

BROWN RICE

Portion out what you need in
Ziploc bags for Days 15 and 17

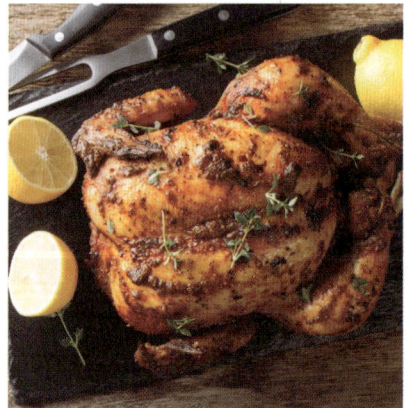

ROTISSERIE CHICKEN

Pull and shred rotisserie chicken for
Caprese Chicken Pasta (p. 122)

MEAL PLAN
DAY 15

BREAKFAST
Easiest-Ever Bagels
(p. 114)

SNACK
1 cup cubed honeydew
or other melon, ½ oz
walnuts (about 7 to 8
halves), and 1 part-skim
cheese stick

LUNCH
Crunchy Chicken Salad
(p. 117)

SNACK
2 Almond and Maple
Energy Bites (p. 118)

DINNER
Pork, Pineapple, and
Red Onion Kebabs
(p. 121) + ½ cup cooked
brown rice

WATER

MOVEMENT Y ☐ N ☐

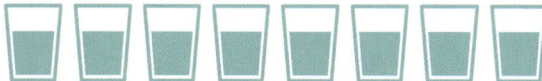

ACTIVITY	DURATION	INTENSITY

SLEEP

BEDTIME	WAKE UP

MOOD

☺ ☻ ☹

MEAL PLAN
DAY 16

↓ **FASTING DAY**

LUNCH
Caprese Chicken Pasta
🔪 (p. 122) + ⅔ cup
pineapple cubes

SNACK
Apple-Cinnamon Yogurt
(p. 125)

SNACK
Easiest-Ever Bagels
🥯 with 2 Tbsp creamy
peanut butter

DINNER
Wild Salmon Salad
(p. 126)

WATER

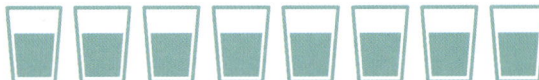

MOVEMENT Y ☐ N ☐

ACTIVITY	DURATION	INTENSITY

SLEEP

BEDTIME	WAKE UP

MOOD

☺ ☻ ☹

MEAL PLAN
DAY 17

BREAKFAST
Cheesy Avocado
Omelet (p. 46)

SNACK
Berry Protein
Smoothie: In a blender
or food processor,
combine 1 cup frozen
mixed berries, 1 cup
unsweetened almond
milk, ½ cup plain nonfat
yogurt, and 1 scoop
protein powder. Add ice,
if desired. Cover and
blend until smooth.

LUNCH
Crunchy Turkey Salad 🥤
+ 1 cup cubed honeydew
or other melon

SNACK
2 Almond Maple Energy
Bites 🗩

DINNER
Seared Coconut-Lime
Chicken with Snap Pea
Slaw + ½ cup cooked
brown rice 🖌

WATER

MOVEMENT Y ☐ N ☐

ACTIVITY	DURATION	INTENSITY

SLEEP

BEDTIME	WAKE UP

MOOD

☺ ☺ ☹

109

MEAL PLAN
DAY 18

LUNCH
Wild Salmon Salad 🥗
+ ⅔ cup pineapple cubes

SNACK
Cheesy Bagel 🔪: Preheat oven to 400°F. Split one Easiest-Ever Bagel and place on baking sheet. Top each half evenly with ½ cup part-skim shredded mozzarella cheese. Bake 7 min. or until cheese melts and bagel is toasty. Serve with marinara sauce for dipping, if desired.

SNACK
1 cup cubed honeydew or other melon, ½ oz walnuts (about 7 to 8 halves), and 1 part-skim cheese stick

DINNER
Peanut Sauce Soba with Crispy Tofu (p. 130)

WATER

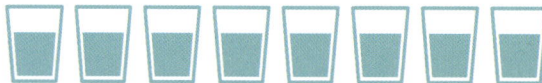

MOVEMENT   Y ☐ N ☐

ACTIVITY	DURATION	INTENSITY

SLEEP

BEDTIME	WAKE UP

MOOD

☺ ☺ ☹

MEAL PLAN
DAY 19

BREAKFAST
Avocado Everything Bagel 🔪: Split and toast one Easiest-Ever Bagel. In a small bowl, cube and mash ½ small avocado. Spread over cut sides of toasted bagel. Sprinkle with Everything Bagel seasoning.

SNACK
1 cup cubed honeydew or other melon + 1 part-skim cheese stick

LUNCH
Pork, Pineapple, and Red Onion Kebabs ♨ + ½ cup cooked brown rice 🔪

SNACK
Apple-Cinnamon Yogurt (p. 125)

DINNER
Baked Halibut with Potatoes and Brussels Sprouts (p. 133)

WATER

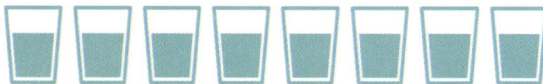

MOVEMENT Y ☐ N ☐

ACTIVITY	DURATION	INTENSITY

SLEEP

BEDTIME	WAKE UP

MOOD

🙂 😐 🙁

MEAL PLAN
DAY 20

↓

FASTING DAY

LUNCH
Peanut Sauce Soba with Crispy Tofu ⛉

SNACK
Berry Protein Smoothie: In a blender or food processor, combine 1 cup frozen mixed berries, 1 cup unsweetened almond milk, ½ cup plain nonfat yogurt, and 1 scoop protein powder. Add ice, if desired. Cover and blend until smooth.

SNACK
1 part-skim cheese stick

DINNER
Caprese Chicken Pasta ⛉ + Simple salad: Toss 1½ cups baby spinach or other leafy green with 2 Tbsp vinaigrette.

WATER

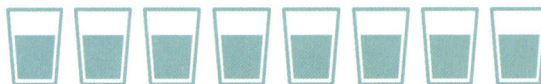

MOVEMENT Y ☐ N ☐

ACTIVITY	DURATION	INTENSITY

SLEEP

BEDTIME	WAKE UP

MOOD

🙂 😐 🙁

112

MEAL PLAN
DAY 21

BREAKFAST
Oatmeal with Greens, Tomato, and Egg (p. 134)

SNACK
1 cup cubed honeydew or other melon, ½ oz walnuts (about 7 to 8 halves), and 1 part-skim cheese stick

LUNCH
Seared Coconut-Lime Chicken with Snap Pea Slaw + ½ cup cooked brown rice

SNACK
Berry Protein Smoothie: In a blender or food processor, combine 1 cup frozen mixed berries, 1 cup unsweetened almond milk, ½ cup plain nonfat yogurt, and 1 scoop protein powder. Add ice, if desired. Cover and blend until smooth.

DINNER
Baked Halibut with Potatoes and Brussels Sprouts

WATER

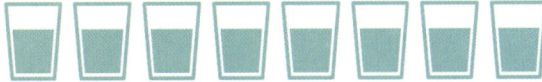

MOVEMENT Y ☐ N ☐

ACTIVITY	DURATION	INTENSITY

SLEEP

BEDTIME	WAKE UP

MOOD

☺ ☻ ☹

EASIEST-EVER BAGELS

ACTIVE **20 MIN.**
TOTAL **50 MIN.**
MAKES **8**

2   cups self-rising flour, plus more for dusting
2   cups plain Greek yogurt
1   large egg, beaten
    Sesame seeds, for topping
    Poppy seeds, for topping
    Onion flakes, for topping
    Everything seasoning, for topping

DIRECTIONS

1. Heat oven to 350°F. Line a baking sheet with parchment paper.

2. In a bowl, combine flour and yogurt until dough starts to form. Turn out dough onto a lightly floured surface and knead 2 min.

3. Divide into 8 parts. Roll each piece of dough into a 1-in.-thick log (about 9 in. long) and pinch ends together to form a circle. Place on prepared baking sheet.

4. Brush tops of bagels with egg, then sprinkle with desired toppings. Bake until golden brown, 28 to 35 min.

NUTRITION

PER BAGEL 185 cal, 10 g pro, 27 g carb, 1 g fiber, 2.5 g sugars (0 g added sugars), 4 g fat (2 g sat fat), 32 mg chol, 415 mg sodium

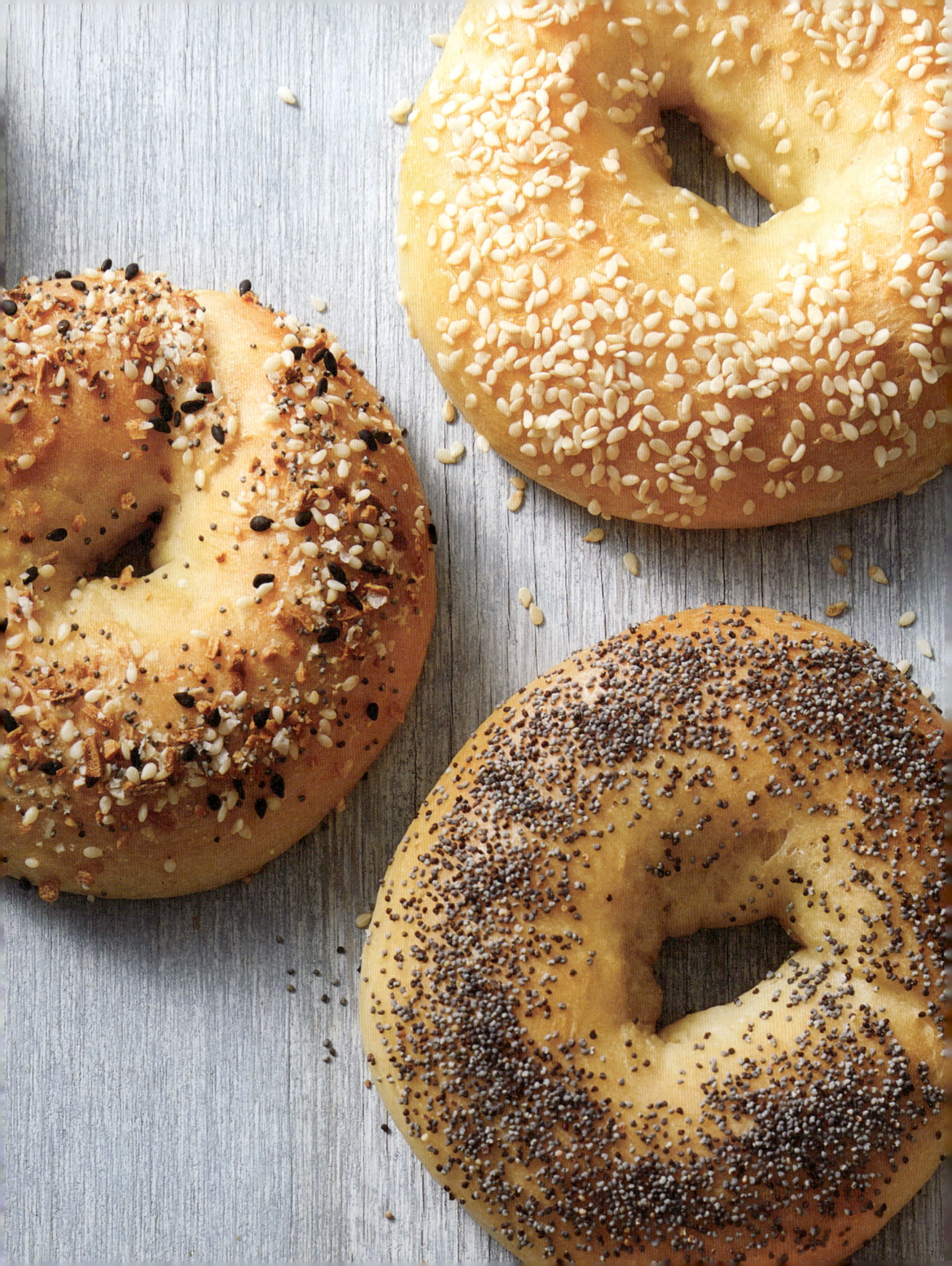

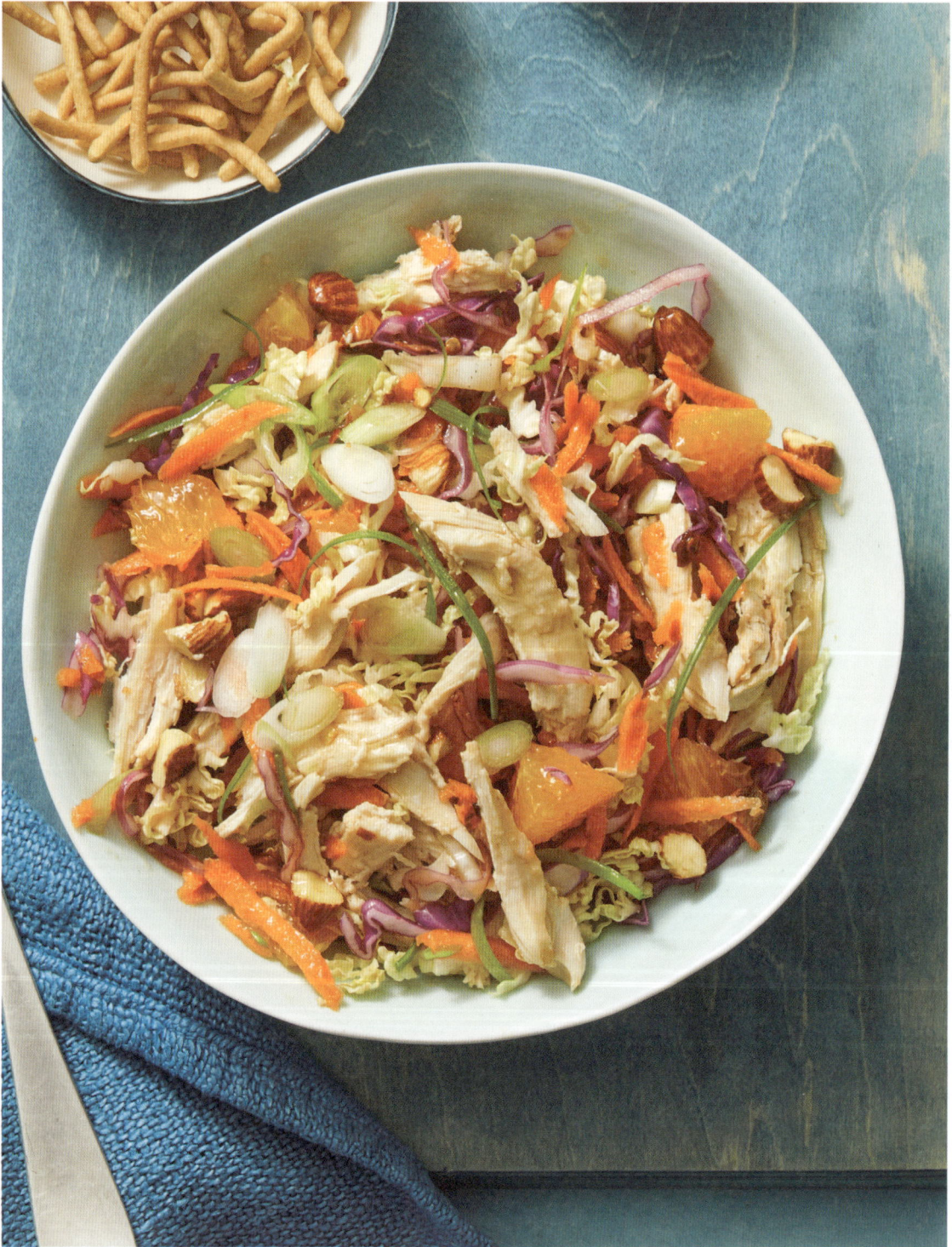

CRUNCHY CHICKEN SALAD

ACTIVE **15 MIN.**
TOTAL **15 MIN.**
SERVES **2**

1½   Tbsp toasted sesame oil
1   Tbsp rice vinegar
½   Tbsp fresh lime juice
1   tsp brown sugar
¼   tsp red pepper flakes
     Kosher salt
½   Napa cabbage, halved and thinly sliced (about 8 cups)
⅛   small red cabbage, thinly sliced (about 1 cup)
1½   cups shredded rotisserie chicken
2   scallions, thinly sliced
1   Cara Cara orange, segmented and cut into pieces
1   medium carrot, coarsely grated
¼   cup crunchy chow mein noodles
¼   cup roasted almonds

DIRECTIONS

1. In large bowl, whisk together toasted sesame oil, rice vinegar, lime juice, brown sugar, red pepper, and ¼ salt.

2. Toss with Napa cabbage, red cabbage, turkey breast, scallions, oranges, and carrot.

3. Serve topped with crunchy chow mein noodles and roasted almonds.

NUTRITION

PER SERVING 490 cal, 41 g pro, 35 g carb, 9 g fiber, 15.5 g sugars (2 g added sugars), 21.5 g fat (2.5 g sat fat), 85 mg chol, 525 mg sodium

ALMOND AND MAPLE ENERGY BITES

ACTIVE **20 MIN.**
TOTAL **50 MIN.**
MAKES **10 TO 12**

¼   **cup almond butter**
2   **Tbsp maple syrup**
½   **Tbsp chia seeds**
¼   **tsp pure vanilla extract**
    Kosher salt
½   **cup old-fashioned oats, toasted**
¼   **cup bittersweet chocolate chips**

DIRECTIONS

1. In a bowl, combine almond butter, maple syrup, chia seeds, vanilla extract, and a pinch of salt. Fold in oats, then chocolate chips. Refrigerate 30 min.

2. Shape mixture into 1-in. balls (about 1 heaping Tbsp each). Store in an airtight container up to 2 weeks or freeze up to 3 months.

NUTRITION
PER BITE 90 cal, 2 g pro, 9 g carb, 2 g fiber, 4.5 g sugars (4 g added sugars), 6 g fat (2 g sat fat), 0 mg chol, 5 mg sodium

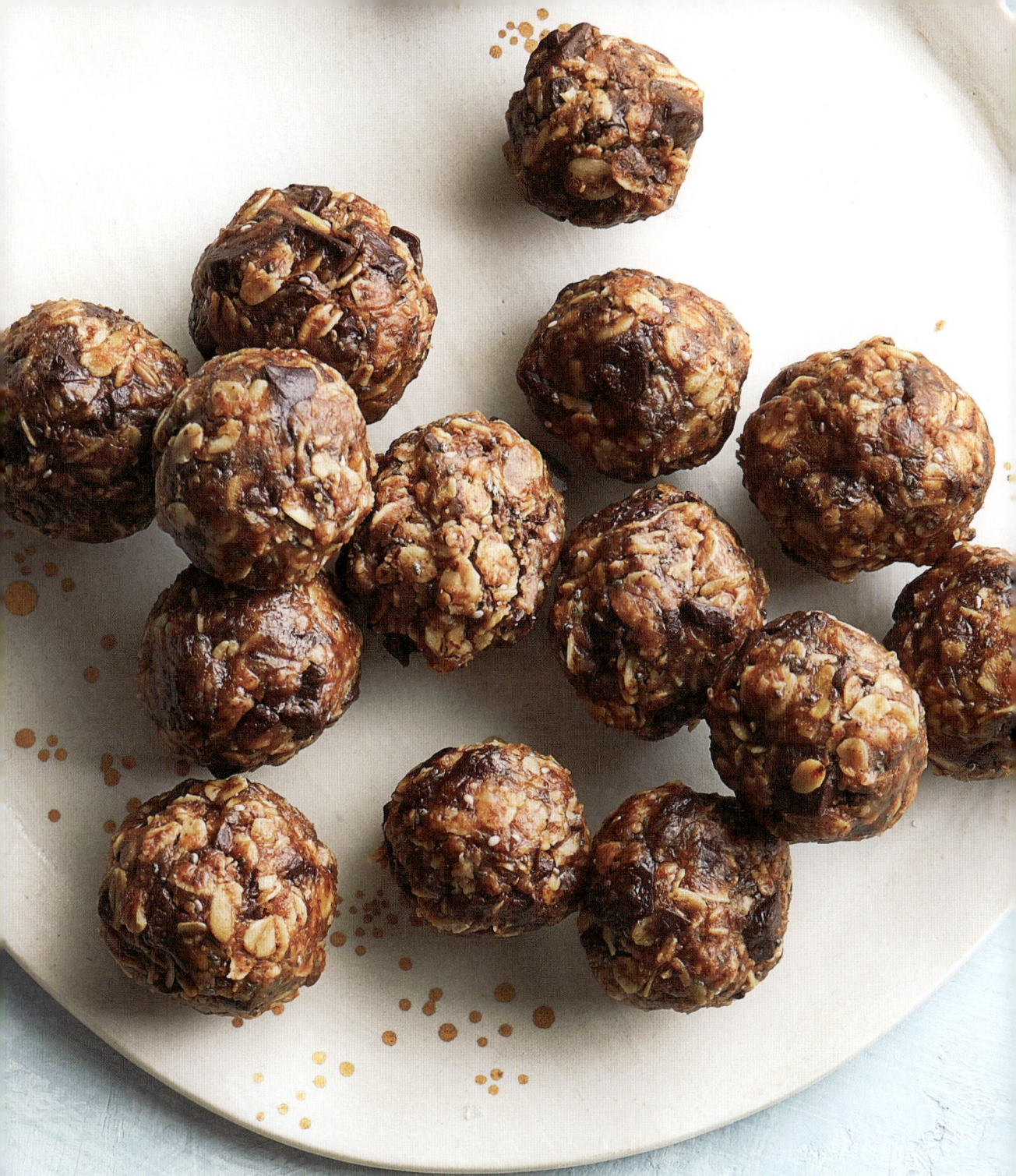

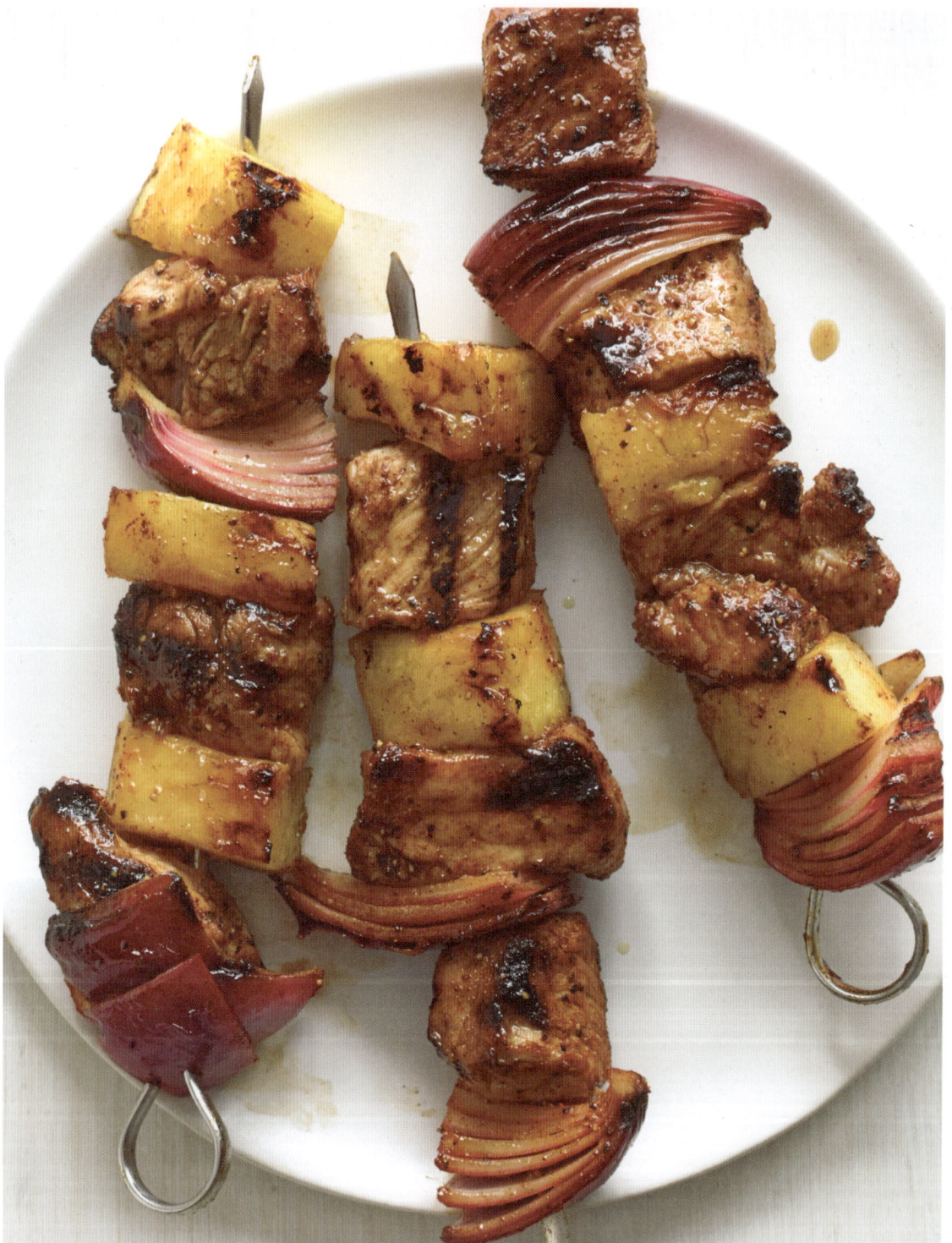

PORK, PINEAPPLE, AND RED ONION KEBABS

ACTIVE **20 MIN.**
TOTAL **20 MIN.**
SERVES **2**

½   **Tbsp brown sugar**
½   **tsp chili powder**
¼   **tsp ground cumin**
½   **Tbsp plus 1 tsp olive oil, divided**
     Kosher salt and pepper
¾   **lb pork loin, cut into 1-in. pieces**
½   **medium red onion**
¼   **small pineapple, cored and cut into 1-in. pieces**

DIRECTIONS

1. Heat grill to medium-high. In a bowl, combine brown sugar, chili powder, ground cumin, 1 tsp olive oil, and ¼ each salt and pepper.

2. Add pork loin and toss to combine.

3. Cut red onion into eight wedges, then cut each wedge in half. In a bowl, toss onion and pineapple with ½ Tbsp olive oil.

4. Thread pork, onion, and pineapple, onto skewers and grill, turning occasionally, until pork is cooked through, 8 to 10 min.

NUTRITION
PER SERVING 420 cal, 35 g pro, 18 g carb, 1 g fiber, 12.5 g sugars (3.5 g added sugars), 23 g fat (7.5 g sat fat), 99 mg chol, 345 mg sodium

CAPRESE CHICKEN PASTA

ACTIVE **5 MIN.**
TOTAL **20 MIN.**
SERVES **2**

4	oz whole-grain penne (about 2 cups cooked)
1	cup shredded rotisserie or cooked chicken (light and/or dark meat)
1	pt cherry tomatoes, halved
2	oz fresh mozzarella pearls
2	Tbsp olive oil
2	Tbsp balsamic vinegar
⅓	cup thinly sliced fresh basil
¼	tsp ground black pepper

DIRECTIONS

1. Cook the pasta per pkg. directions. Drain and transfer to a medium bowl.

2. Toss together the penne, chicken, tomatoes, and mozzarella.

3. In a separate bowl, whisk together the olive oil, vinegar, basil, and pepper. Toss the dressing with the pasta.

NUTRITION
PER SERVING 510 cal, 35 g pro, 49 g carb, 7 g fiber, 8 g sugars (0 g added sugars), 22 g fat (5 g sat fat), 80 mg chol, 320 mg sodium

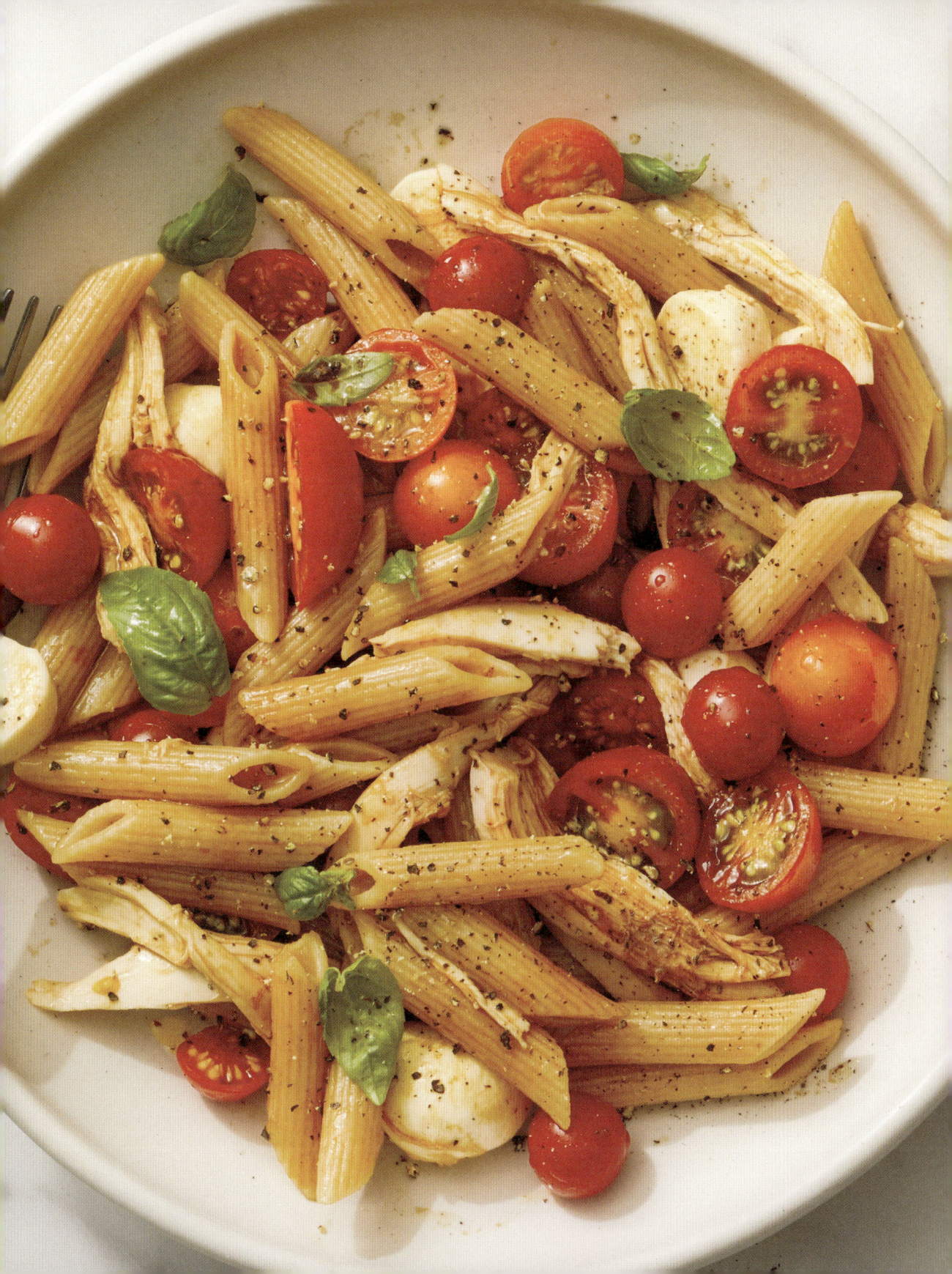

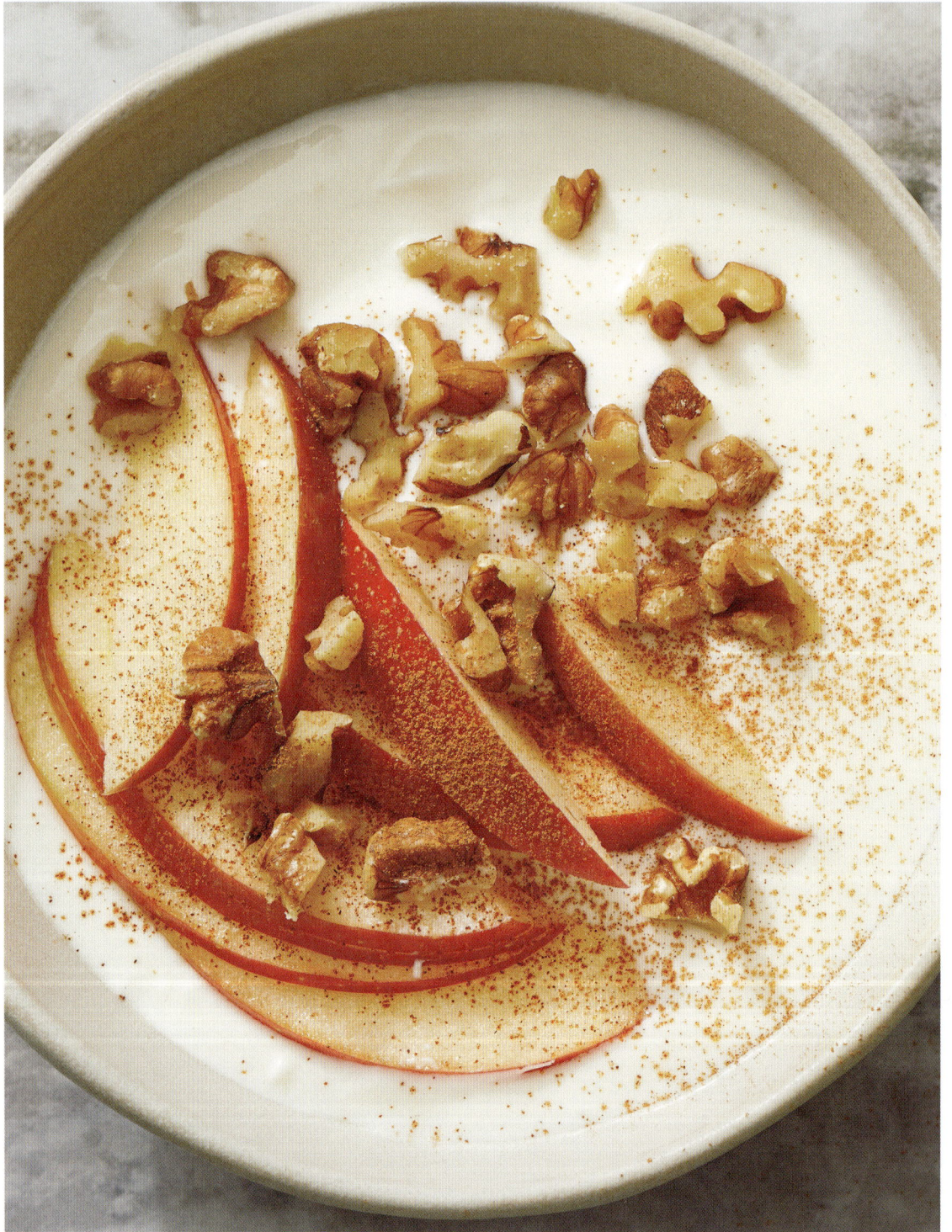

APPLE-CINNAMON YOGURT

ACTIVE **1 MIN.**
TOTAL **2 MIN.**
SERVES **1**

1	small apple, cored and chopped
2	Tbsp chopped walnuts
1	tsp honey (optional)
¼	tsp ground cinnamon
½	cup fat-free plain yogurt

DIRECTIONS
Place the apple and walnuts in a bowl. Top with the honey, if using, and cinnamon. Microwave on high for 1 minute, or until warmed. Top with the yogurt.

NUTRITION
PER SERVING 240 cal, 10 g pro, 32 g carb, 5 g fiber, 25 g sugars (0 g added sugars), 10 g fat (1 g sat fat), 2 mg chol, 95 mg sodium

WILD SALMON SALAD

2	4-oz skinless wild Alaskan salmon fillets
	Kosher salt and pepper
1	Tbsp balsamic vinegar
1	tsp olive oil
½	pt grape tomatoes, halved
1	scallions, thinly sliced
2.5	oz mixed baby greens
½	avocado, sliced
¼	cup slivered almonds, toasted

DIRECTIONS

1. Heat oven to 375°F. Season salmon with ¼ tsp each salt and pepper, place on a rimmed baking sheet, and roast until opaque throughout, 10 to 12 min.

2. Meanwhile, in a large bowl, whisk together vinegar, oil, and a pinch of salt and pepper. Toss with tomatoes, then fold in scallions followed by greens.

3. Serve with salmon and avocado and sprinkle with almonds.

NUTRITION
PER SERVING 340 cal, 28 g pro, 13 g carb, 7 g fiber, 4.5 g sugars (0 g added sugars), 20.5 g fat (3 g sat fat), 72 mg chol, 350 mg sodium

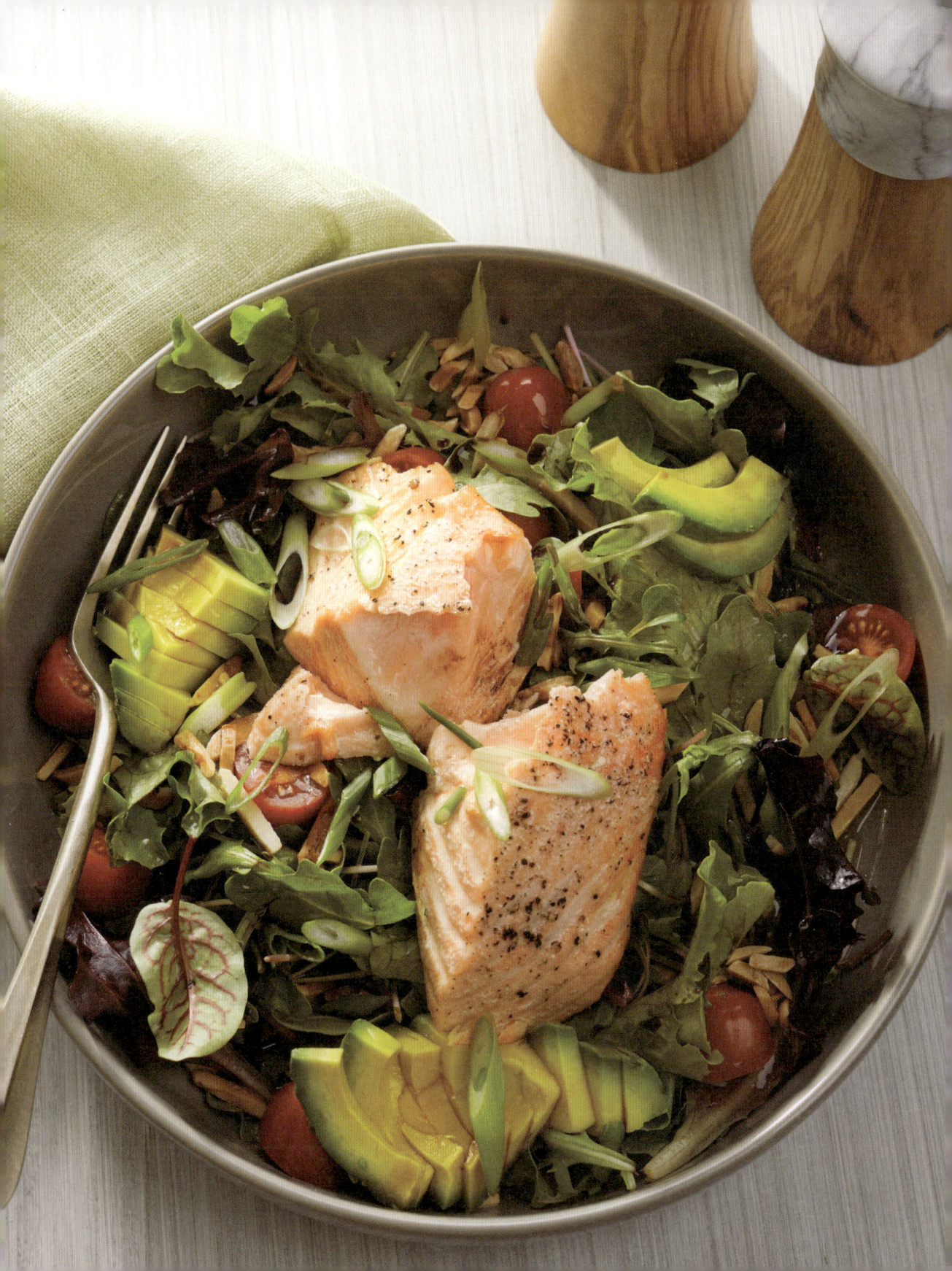

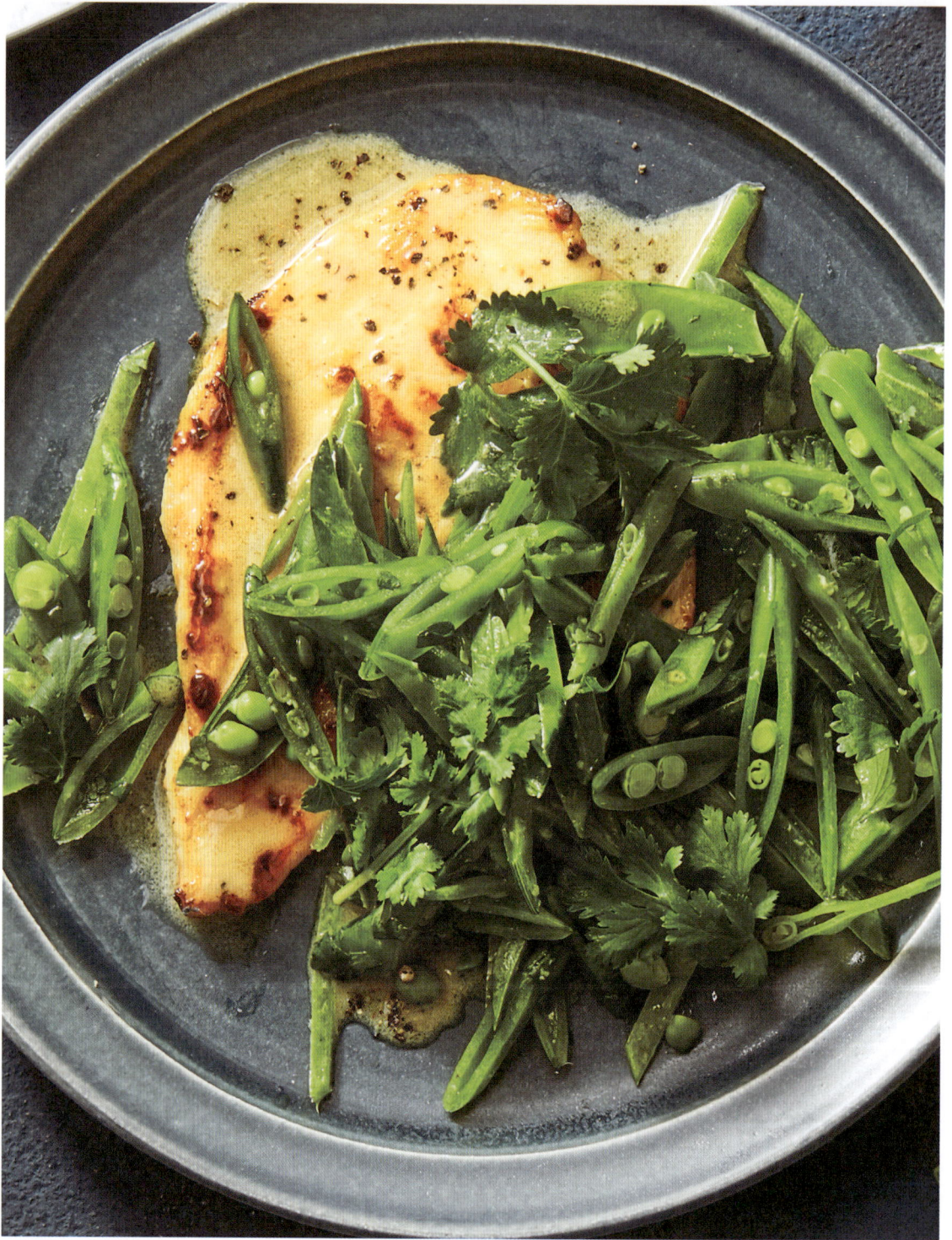

SEARED COCONUT-LIME CHICKEN WITH SNAP PEA SLAW

ACTIVE **45 MIN.**
TOTAL **45 MIN.**
SERVES **2**

1	Tbsp toasted sesame oil
½	Tbsp grated fresh ginger
1½	Tbsp fresh lime juice, divided
	Kosher salt and pepper
5	oz snap peas, string removed and thinly sliced
2	oz snow peas, thinly sliced
1	scallions, thinly sliced
1	8-oz boneless, skinless chicken breasts
½	Tbsp olive oil
1	Tbsp coconut cream
¼	cup cilantro

DIRECTIONS

1. In a medium bowl, whisk together sesame oil, ginger, ¾ Tbsp lime juice and ¼ tsp salt. Add snap peas, snow peas, and scallions, and toss to combine.

2. Cut chicken breast horizontally in half to make 2 thin cutlets, then pound to ¼-in. thick. Heat oil in a large skillet on medium-high. Season chicken with ¼ tsp each salt and pepper and cook in batches until golden brown and cooked through, about 2 min. per side. Transfer chicken to plates as it is cooked. Remove pan from heat and stir in coconut cream and remaining ¾ Tbsp lime juice, scraping up any browned bits. Spoon over chicken on plates.

3. Fold cilantro into pea mixture and serve on top of chicken.

NUTRITION
PER SERVING 290 cal, 29 g pro, 10 g carb, 3 g fiber, 9 g sugars (0 g added sugars), 15 g fat (3.5 g sat fat), 85 mg chol, 540 mg sodium

PEANUT SAUCE SOBA WITH CRISPY TOFU

ACTIVE **25 MIN**.
TOTAL **35 MIN**.
SERVES **2**

1	**12.3-oz packages extra-firm tofu, drained**
1½	**Tbsp canola oil**
1	**tsp grated garlic, divided**
1¼	**Tbsp low-sodium soy sauce, divided**
1½	**Tbsp natural smooth peanut butter**
½	**Tbsp agave or honey**
½	**Tbsp fresh lime juice**
2	**Tbsp hot water**
⅛	**tsp grated ginger**
½	**tsp sriracha**
½	**Tbsp toasted sesame oil**
⅓	**cup cornstarch**
4	**oz soba noodles, cooked per package directions**
3	**cups baby spinach**

DIRECTIONS

1. Pat tofu dry with paper towels and cut into ¾-in. cubes.

2. In a small bowl, whisk together canola oil, half of garlic, and ½ Tbsp soy sauce. Transfer one-third to a small baking dish, coating bottom evenly. Add tofu and pour remaining marinade on top. Gently turn tofu to coat and let sit at room temperature, 45 min.

3. In a medium bowl, combine peanut butter, agave, and lime juice with remaining ¾ Tbsp soy sauce. Gradually whisk in hot water to emulsify. Whisk in ginger, sriracha, sesame oil, and remaining garlic. Set aside.

4. Heat air fryer to 400°F. Carefully dredge marinated tofu in cornstarch, coating evenly and shaking off excess. Add tofu to air fryer basket, spacing apart. Air-fry, shaking basket twice, until golden brown and crisp, 15 to 18 min.

5. Meanwhile, in a large bowl, toss warm soba noodles with baby spinach and peanut sauce. Serve topped with crispy tofu.

NUTRITION
PER SERVING 695 cal, 33 g pro, 79 g carb, 4 g fiber, 5 g sugars (4 g added sugars), 30 g fat (4 g sat fat), 0 mg chol, 300 mg sodium

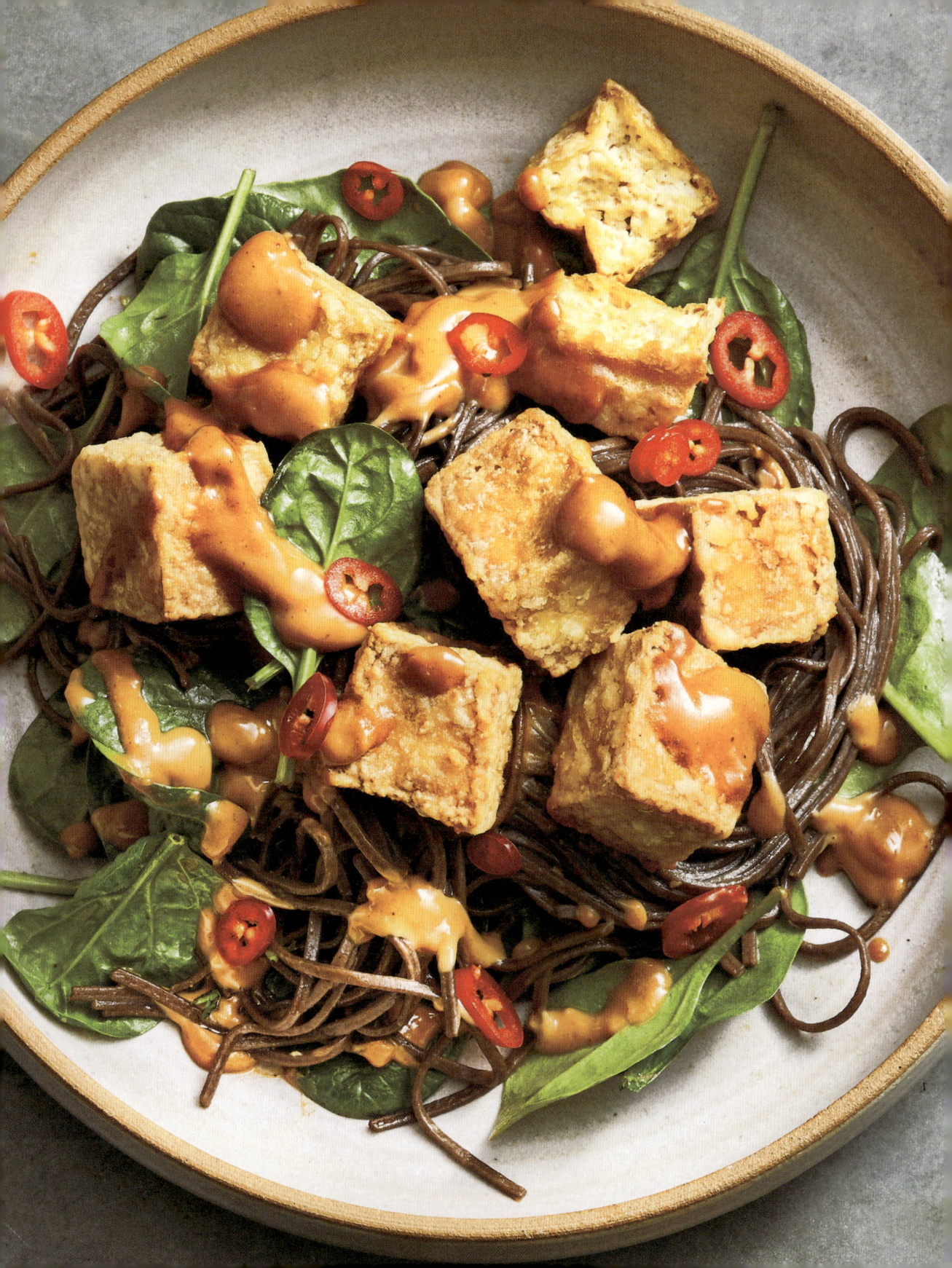

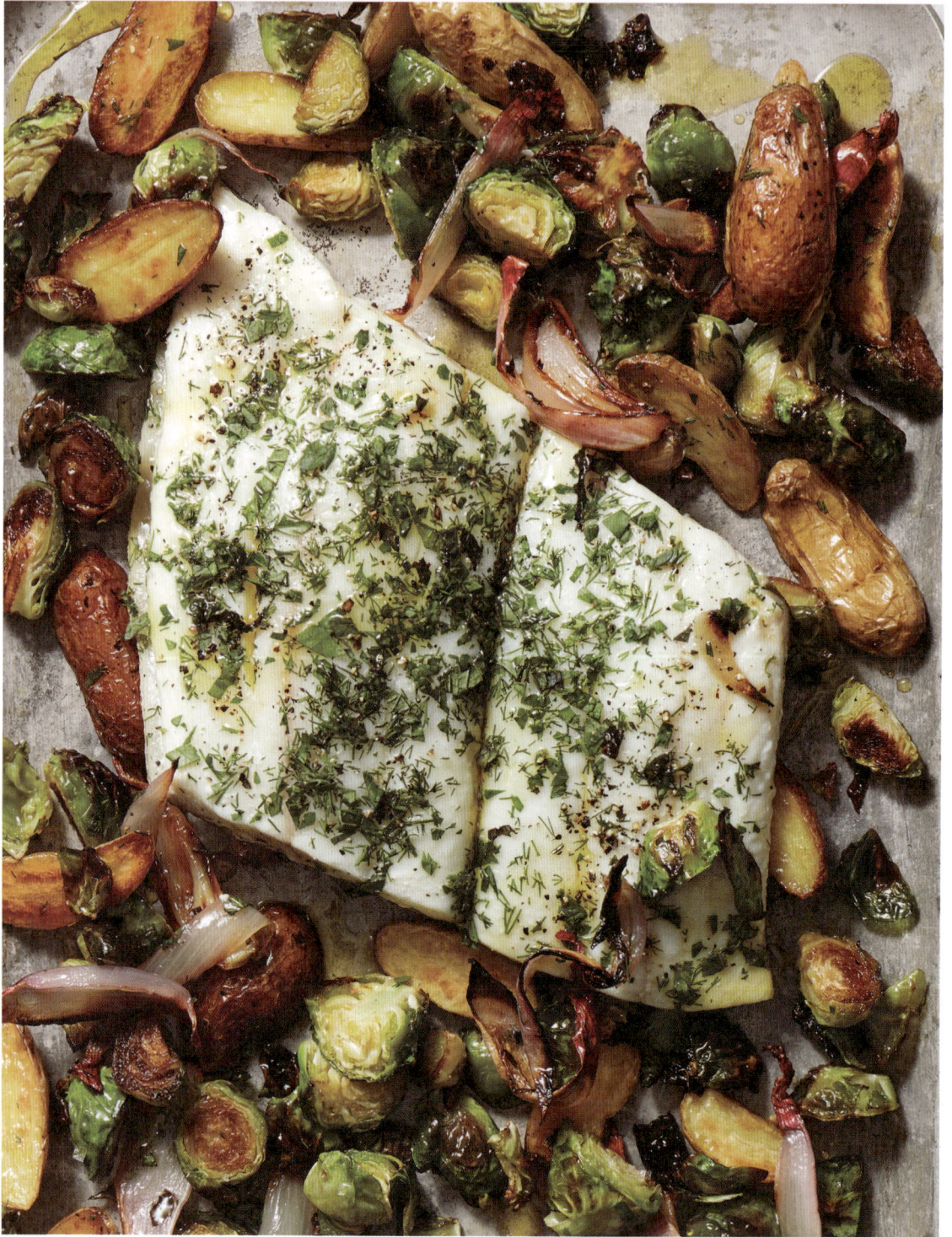

BAKED HALIBUT WITH POTATOES AND BRUSSELS SPROUTS

ACTIVE **20 MIN.**
TOTAL **35 MIN.**
SERVES **2**

1   Tbsp olive oil
1   Tbsp chopped mixed fresh herbs (such as parsley, thyme, and rosemary)
    Kosher salt and pepper
½   lb fingerling potatoes (about 20), halved
½   lb Brussels sprouts (about 10), trimmed and quartered
½   large shallot, cut into wedges
¾   lb halibut fillet

DIRECTIONS

1. Heat oven to 425°F. In a bowl, whisk together oil, herbs, ⅜ tsp salt, and ¼ tsp pepper.

2. On a large rimmed baking sheet, toss potatoes, Brussels sprouts, and shallot with half of oil mixture. Arrange potatoes cut side down; roast 15 min.

3. Remove the pan from oven and set halibut fillet on top of vegetables. Brush halibut with remaining oil mixture and roast until potatoes are golden brown and tender and halibut is opaque throughout, 12 to 15 min. more.

NUTRITION
PER SERVING 370 cal, 40 g pro, 37 g carb, 7 g fiber, 6 g sugars (0 g added sugars), 9 g fat (2 g sat fat), 83 mg chol, 505 mg sodium

OATMEAL WITH GREENS, TOMATO, AND EGG

ACTIVE **10 MIN.**
TOTAL **10 MIN.**
SERVES **1**

¼ **cup quick-cooking steel-cut oats**
   Kosher salt
¼ **cup grape tomatoes, sliced in half**
1 **scallion, thinly sliced**
2 **tsp olive oil**
¾ **cup baby spinach**
   Soft-boiled egg, halved

DIRECTIONS

1. In a small saucepan, bring ¾ cup water to a boil. Add oats and pinch of salt and cook, stirring occasionally, until tender, 5 to 7 min.

2. Meanwhile, in a small bowl, toss tomatoes, scallion, oil, and pinch of salt.

3. Remove oatmeal from heat and fold in spinach to wilt. Transfer to serving bowl, top with tomatoes and egg.

NUTRITION
PER SERVING 250 cal, 10 g pro, 18 g carb, 4 g fiber, 2 g sugars (0 g added sugars), 15 g fat (3 g sat fat), 185 mg chol, 110 mg sodium

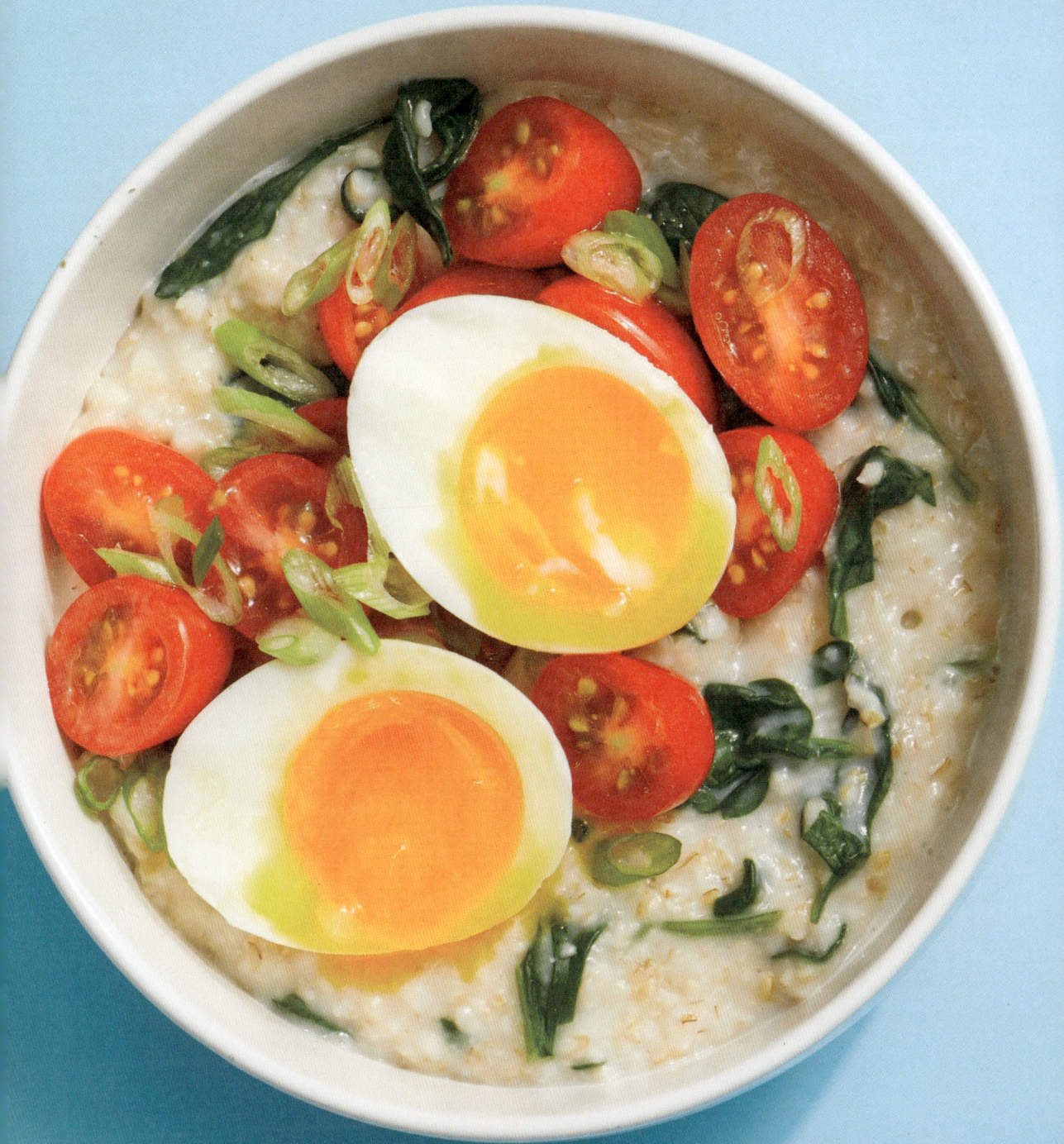

WEEK 4: AT-A-GLANCE

Day 22

BREAKFAST
1 Berry-Quinoa Muffin ⊏⊐ + 2 scrambled eggs

SNACK
Top ¾ cup low-fat, lower-sodium cottage cheese with ⅓ cup blueberries or other berry

LUNCH
Green Goddess Sandwich ✐

SNACK
1 orange, 1 part-skim cheese stick, and 1 oz almonds (approximately 20-22 pieces)

DINNER
Salmon and Asparagus With Snap Pea Salad

Day 23 - FASTING

LUNCH
Green Envy Rice Bowl ✐ + 1 medium orange

SNACK
1 slice toasted whole-grain bread topped with 2 Tbsp almond butter or other nut butter

SNACK
1 serving Curried White Bean Dip ⊏⊐ + 1½ oz whole-wheat pita chips (about 13 chips)

DINNER
Grilled Chicken Skewers and Kale Caesar

Day 24

BREAKFAST
Curry-Avocado Crispy Egg Toast

SNACK
⅔ cup blueberries or other berry

LUNCH
Green Goddess Sandwich ✐

SNACK
1 apple with 1 Tbsp almond butter or other nut butter

DINNER
Cod with Orange Leek Couscous + Roasted Asparagus

Day 25 - FASTING

LUNCH
Green Envy Rice Bowl ⊎

SNACK
1 slice whole-grain bread, toasted, topped with mashed avocado (approximately ½ of a small avocado

SNACK
¾ cup vanilla Greek yogurt, ⅓ cup blueberries, and 2 Tbsp chopped walnuts

DINNER
Homemade Turkey Sausage, Fennel, and Arugula with Chickpea Rigatoni + leftover Roasted Asparagus

Day 26

BREAKFAST
1 Berry-Quinoa Muffin ⊏⊐ + 2 scrambled eggs

SNACK
Top ¾ cup low-fat, lower-sodium cottage cheese with ⅓ cup blueberries or other berry

LUNCH
Cod with Orange Leek Couscous ⊎

SNACK
Curried White Bean Dip ⊏⊐ + ½ seedless cucumber, cut into slices

DINNER
Chicken with Fried Cauliflower Rice + Quick Roasted Broccoli

Day 27 - FASTING

LUNCH
Grilled Chicken Skewers and Kale Caesar ⊎

SNACK
Avocado-Egg Toast

SNACK
Green Pineapple Coconut Smoothie

DINNER
Homemade Turkey Sausage, Fennel, and Arugula with Chickpea Rigatoni ⊎ + Simple salad

Day 28

BREAKFAST
Green Pineapple Coconut Smoothie ⊎ + 1 oz dry-roasted almonds (approximately 20 to 22)

SNACK
Top ¾ cup low-fat, lower-sodium cottage cheese with ⅓ cup blueberries or other berry

LUNCH
Chicken with Fried Cauliflower Rice ⊎

SNACK
1 Berry-Quinoa Muffin ⊏⊐ + 1 part-skim mozzarella pint

DINNER
Sheet Pan Chicken Tikka with Cauliflower and Chickpeas

⊏⊐ **Fully prepped**

✐ **Partially prepped**

⊎ **Leftover**

SHOPPING LIST

PRODUCE

- 2 cups blueberries
- 1 6-oz container raspberries
- 2½ oranges
- 1 lime
- 2 bunches asparagus (about 2 lb total)
- 3 oz sugar snap peas
- 1 Tbsp tarragon
- 2¼ avocado
- 8 cloves garlic
- 5 lemons
- 1 onion
- ¼ red onion
- ¼ lb Brussels sprouts
- ¼ lb cremini mushrooms
- 4½ cups baby kale
- 1 apple
- 2 Tbsp basil
- 4 Tbsp chives
- 2½ cups salad greens
- ¾ seedless cucumber
- ½ cup sprouts
- 4 Tbsp cilantro
- ½ leek
- ½ fennel bulb
- 2 cups baby arugula
- 1½ cups broccoli florets
- 2 cups baby spinach
- 1 banana
- 1 red bell pepper
- 1 small carrot
- 6 oz carrots
- 2 scallions
- 2 cups cauliflower "rice"
- ¼ head cauliflower

MEAT & SEAFOOD

- 2 6-oz skinless salmon fillets
- 1 cup shredded rotisserie or cooked chicken
- ¾ lb skinless, boneless chicken breast
- 2 5-oz cod fillets
- ½ lb lean ground turkey
- 2 chicken legs

REFRIGERATOR & DAIRY

- 1 dozen eggs
- ½ cup plain whole-milk yogurt
- 2 Tbsp whole milk
- 2¼ cups low-fat, lower-sodium cottage cheese
- 2 part-skim cheese stick
- ½ cup kimchi
- 2 Tbsp grated Parmesan
- ¾ cup low-fat vanilla Green yogurt
- 2½ Tbsp grated Pecorino Romano

- 2 Tbsp plain low-fat yogurt

FROZEN

- 1 cup frozen pineapple chunks
- ½ cup frozen peas

BREAD & BAKERY

- 8 slices whole-grain bread
- 1½ oz whole-grain pita chips
- 4 slices baguette

PANTRY

- 6 Tbsp all-purpose flour
- ½ cup almond flour
- 2 Tbsp white quinoa
- ½ tsp baking powder
- ½ tsp ground cinnamon
- ¼ tsp ground ginger
- ¼ tsp baking soda
- 2½ Tbsp honey
- 2 oz dry-roasted almonds
- 3 Tbsp almond butter or other nut butter
- 17 Tbsp olive oil
- 2¼ tsp curry powder
- 1 15-oz can white beans
- ½ tsp ground cumin

- ½ tsp smoked paprika
- 1 tsp sweet paprika
- 1⅛ tsp garlic powder
- 1 cup brown rice
- 2 Tbsp tahini
- 2 Tbsp apple cider vinegar
- 1 tsp rice vinegar
- ½ tsp miso paste
- 2 Tbsp Dijon mustard
- 2½ Tbsp mayonnaise
- ½ cup couscous
- 2 Tbsp chopped walnuts
- ½ tsp red pepper flakes
- 6 oz chickpea or other legume-based pasta
- 1 Tbsp fennel seeds
- ½ tsp Everything Bagel seasoning
- 1 cup canned light coconut milk
- 2½ tsp grapeseed oil
- 1 Tbsp low-sodium soy sauce
- ½ cup jarred tikka masala sauce
- ½ cup canned chickpeas
- ½ tsp garam masala
- 2½ Tbsp roasted salted pistachios

MEAL PREP DAY

Make it easy by partially prepping the day before you start your week.

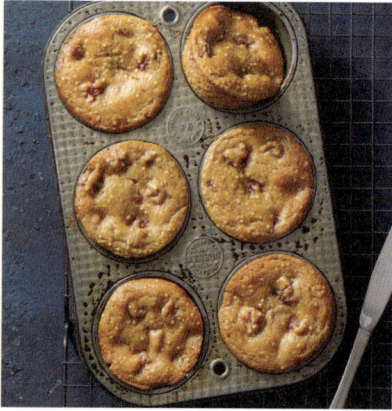

BERRY-QUINOA MUFFINS (P. 146)

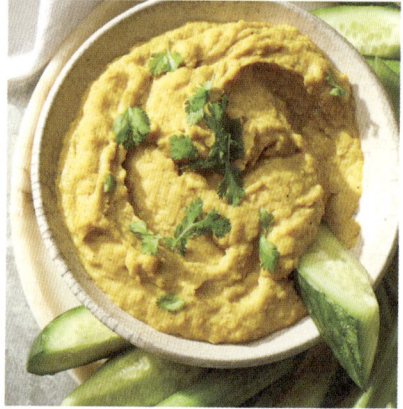

CURRIED WHITE BEAN DIP (P. 154)

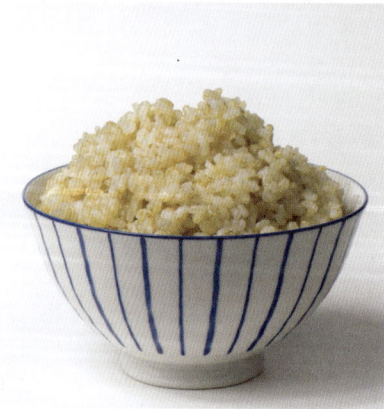

BROWN RICE

Cook 1 cup for Green Envy Rice Bowls

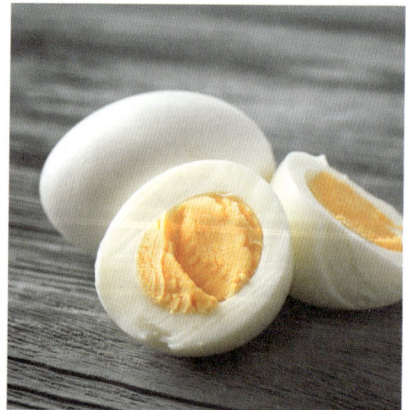

HARD-BOILED EGGS

Boil 2 eggs for Green Goddess Sandwiches

MEAL PLAN
DAY 22

BREAKFAST
1 Berry Quinoa Muffin 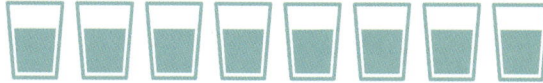 (p. 146) +
2 scrambled eggs

SNACK
Top ¾ cup low-fat, lower-sodium cottage cheese with ⅓ cup blueberries or other berry

LUNCH
Green Goddess Sandwich (p. 149)

SNACK
1 orange, 1 part-skim cheese stick, and 1 oz almonds (approximately 20 to 22 pieces)

DINNER
Salmon and Asparagus With Snap Pea Salad (p. 150)

WATER

MOVEMENT Y ☐ N ☐

ACTIVITY	DURATION	INTENSITY

SLEEP

BEDTIME	WAKE UP

MOOD

☺ ☻ ☹

MEAL PLAN
DAY 23

LUNCH
Green Envy Rice Bowl 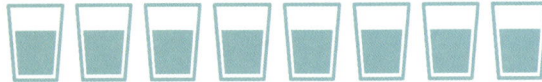 (p. 153) + 1 medium orange

SNACK
1 slice toasted whole-grain bread topped with 2 Tbsp almond butter or other nut butter

SNACK
1 serving Curried White Bean Dip 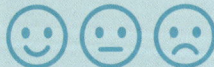 (p. 154) + 1½ oz whole-wheat pita chips (about 13 chips)

DINNER
Grilled Chicken Skewers and Kale Caesar (p. 157)

WATER

MOVEMENT   Y ☐ N ☐

ACTIVITY	DURATION	INTENSITY

SLEEP

BEDTIME	WAKE UP

MOOD

☺ ☻ ☹

MEAL PLAN
DAY 24

BREAKFAST
Curry-Avocado Crispy
Egg Toast (p. 158)

SNACK
⅔ cup blueberries or
other berry

LUNCH
Green Goddess
Sandwich 🖊 (p. 149)

SNACK
1 apple with 1 Tbsp
almond butter or other
nut butter

DINNER
Cod with Orange Leek
Couscous (p. 161) +
Roasted Asparagus:
Trim the ends off a 1-lb
bunch of asparagus.
Heat oven to 425°F. Toss
asparagus with
2 Tbsp olive oil, ½ tsp
garlic powder, and
¼ tsp kosher salt.
Spread evenly across a
rimmed baking sheet.
Bake 7 to 9 min. or until
asparagus begins to
turn tender and brown
on edges. Reserve half
for tomorrow's dinner.

WATER

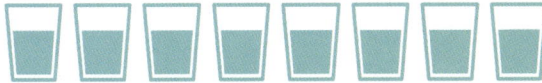

MOVEMENT Y ☐ N ☐

ACTIVITY	DURATION	INTENSITY

SLEEP

BEDTIME	WAKE UP

MOOD

🙂 😐 🙁

MEAL PLAN
DAY 25

LUNCH
Green Envy Rice Bowl

SNACK
1 slice whole-grain bread, toasted, topped with mashed avocado (approximately ½ of a small avocado

SNACK
¾ cup vanilla Greek yogurt, ⅓ cup blueberries, and 2 Tbsp chopped walnuts

DINNER
Homemade Turkey Sausage, Fennel, and Arugula with Chickpea Rigatoni (p. 162) + Roasted Asparagus

WATER

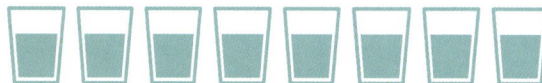

MOVEMENT   Y ☐ N ☐

ACTIVITY	DURATION	INTENSITY

SLEEP

BEDTIME	WAKE UP

MOOD

☺ ☺ ☹

MEAL PLAN
DAY 26

BREAKFAST
1 Berry-Quinoa Muffin
⊂⊐ + 2 scrambled eggs

SNACK
Top ¾ cup low-fat, lower-sodium cottage cheese with ⅓ cup blueberries or other berry

LUNCH
Cod with Orange Leek Couscous ♨

SNACK
1 serving Curried White Bean Dip ⊂⊐ + ½ seedless cucumber, cut into slices

DINNER
Chicken with Fried Cauliflower Rice (p. 165) + Quick Roasted Broccoli: Toss 1½ cups broccoli florets with 1 Tbsp olive oil and ⅛ tsp garlic powder. Bake at 400°F for 9 to 11 min. or until edges start to brown.

WATER

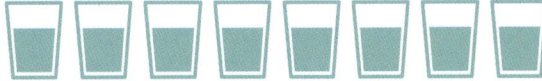

MOVEMENT Y ☐ N ☐

ACTIVITY	DURATION	INTENSITY

SLEEP

BEDTIME	WAKE UP

MOOD

☺ ☺ ☹

MEAL PLAN
DAY 27

↓

FASTING DAY

LUNCH
Grilled Chicken Skewers and Kale Caesar ♨

SNACK
Avocado-Egg Toast: Mash ½ of a small avocado and spread on 1 slice toasted whole-grain bread. Top with a sliced hardboiled egg and sprinkle with Everything Bagel seasoning.

SNACK
Green Pineapple Coconut Smoothie (p. 166)

DINNER
Homemade Turkey Sausages, Fennel, and Arugula with Chickpea Rigatoni ♨ + Simple salad: Toss 1½ cups mixed salad greens with 2 Tbsp vinaigrette.

WATER

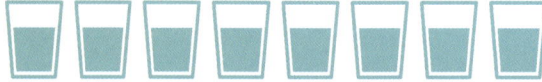

MOVEMENT   Y ☐ N ☐

ACTIVITY	DURATION	INTENSITY

SLEEP

BEDTIME	WAKE UP

MOOD

☺ ☺ ☹

MEAL PLAN
DAY 28

BREAKFAST
Green Pineapple Coconut Smoothie (p. 166) + 1 oz dry-roasted almonds (approximately 20 to 22)

SNACK
Top ¾ cup low-fat, lower-sodium cottage cheese with ⅓ cup blueberries or other berry

LUNCH
Chicken with Fried Cauliflower Rice

SNACK
1 Berry- Quinoa Muffin 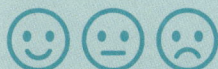 + 1 part-skim mozzarella pint

DINNER
Sheet Pan Chicken Tikka with Cauliflower and Chickpeas (p. 169)

WATER

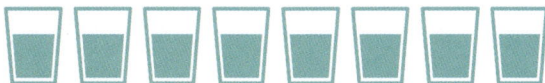

MOVEMENT Y ☐ N ☐

ACTIVITY	DURATION	INTENSITY

SLEEP

BEDTIME	WAKE UP

MOOD

☺ ☐ ☹

145

BERRY-QUINOA MUFFINS

ACTIVE **10 MIN.**
TOTAL **30 MIN.**
MAKES **6**

6	Tbsp all-purpose flour, plus more for dusting
½	cup almond flour
⅛	cup white quinoa (uncooked)
½	tsp baking powder
½	tsp ground cinnamon
¼	tsp ground ginger
¼	tsp baking soda
¼	tsp kosher salt
1	large eggs, beaten
½	cup plain whole-milk yogurt
⅛	cup whole milk
2½	Tbsp honey
1	6-oz container raspberries

DIRECTIONS

1. Heat oven to 325°F. Lightly coat a 6-cup muffin pan with cooking spray and dust with flour.

2. In a large bowl, whisk together flours, quinoa, baking powder, cinnamon, ginger, baking soda, and salt.

3. In a medium bowl, whisk together eggs, yogurt, milk, and honey. Fold egg mixture into flour mixture until just combined, then stir in raspberries.

4. Divide batter among muffin pan cups and bake until toothpick inserted into centers come out clean, 15 to 20 min. Cool in pan 5 min., then transfer to wire rack to cool completely.

NUTRITION

PER MUFFIN 175 cal, 6 g pro, 24 g carb, 4 g fiber, 10.5 g sugars (7.5 g added sugars), 7 g fat (1 g sat fat), 34 mg chol, 205 mg sodium

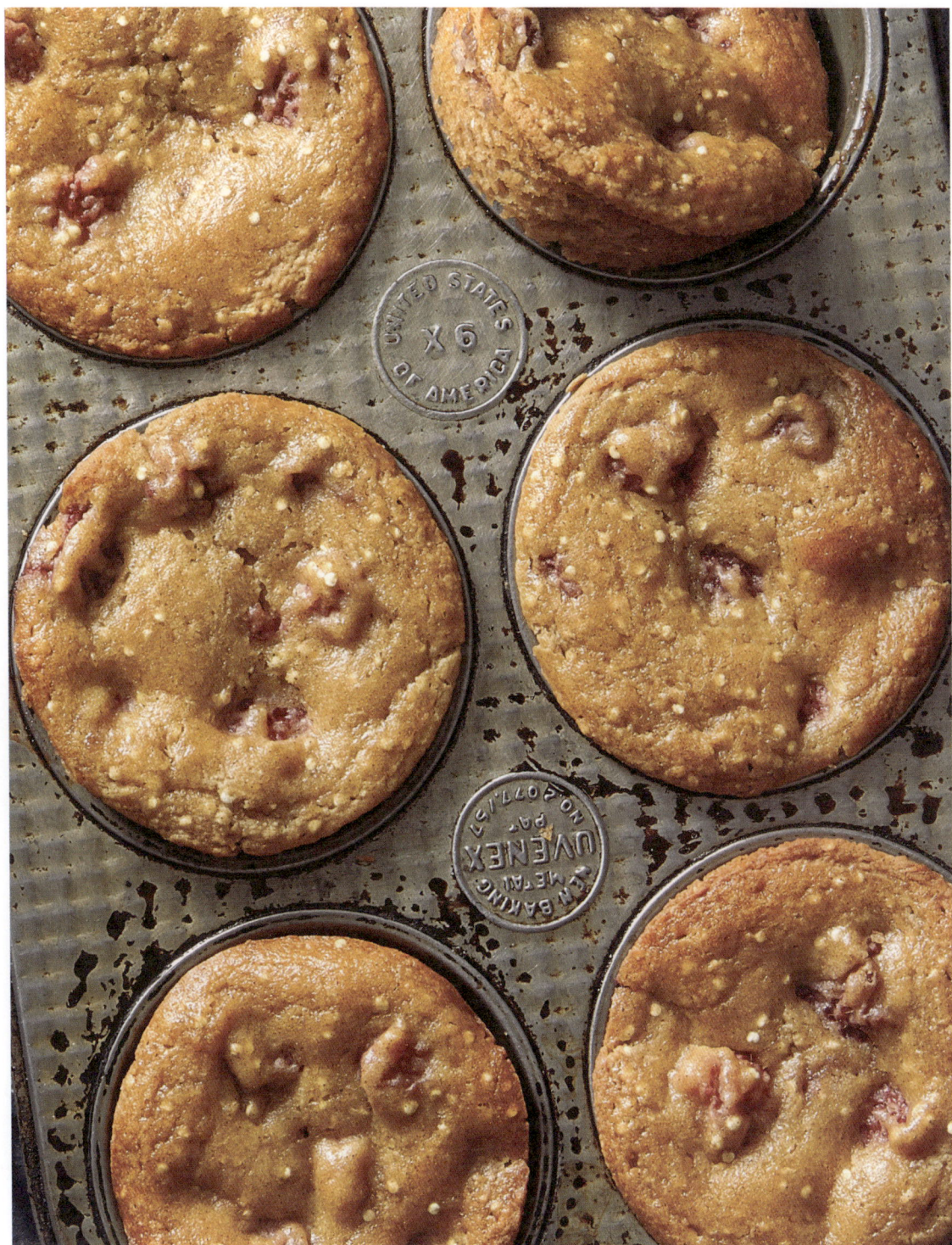

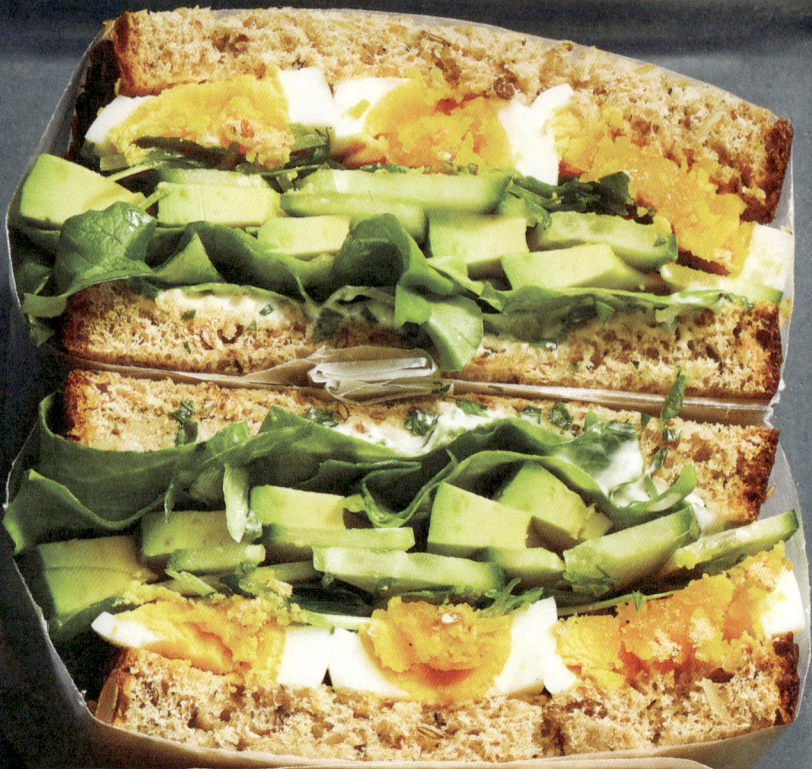

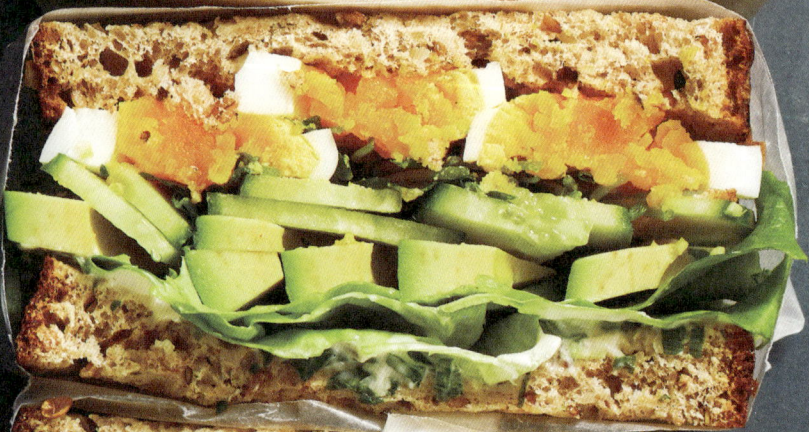

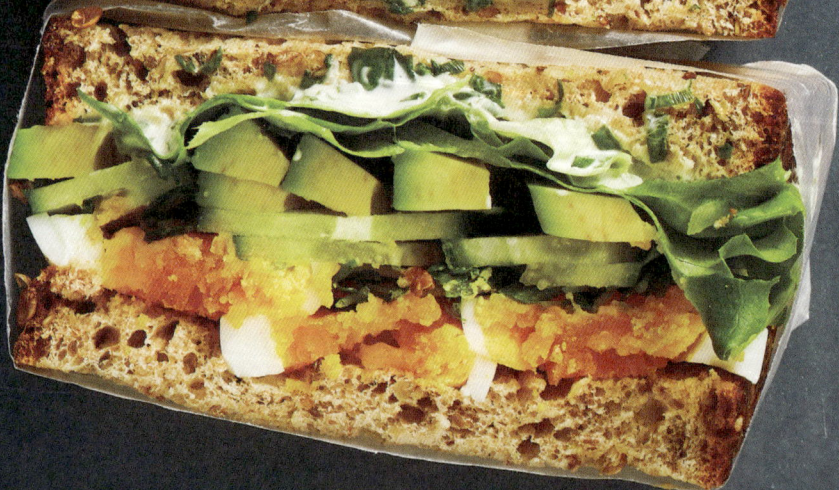

GREEN GODDESS SANDWICHES

ACTIVE **15 MIN.**
TOTAL **15 MIN.**
SERVES **2**

2	large eggs
	Ice water, for cooling
2½	Tbsp mayonnaise
¼	Tbsp lemon juice
¼	small clove garlic, finely grated
	Kosher salt and pepper
2	Tbsp basil, chopped
1	Tbsp chopped chives
4	slices whole-grain bread
1	cup salad greens or favorite lettuce
½	avocado, sliced
¼	seedless cucumber, halved crosswise and thinly slice lengthwise
½	cup sprouts

DIRECTIONS

1. Heat air fryer to 275°F. Place eggs in air-fryer basket and air-fry 15 min. Immediately transfer eggs to a bowl of ice water to cool for a few min., then peel and slice the eggs.

2. Meanwhile, in a small bowl, combine mayonnaise, lemon juice, garlic, and ⅛ tsp each salt and pepper; fold in basil and chives.

3. Spread basil mayonnaise on bread, then create sandwiches with lettuce, avocado, cucumber, sprouts and eggs.

Make-Ahead Eggs: Air-fry or boil eggs, then add to ice water to cool. Refrigerate in shells for up to one week. Peel right before using.

NUTRITION
PER SERVING 435 cal, 16 g pro, 30 g carb, 8 g fiber, 6 g sugars (0 g added sugars), 29 g fat (5.5 g sat fat), 194 mg chol, 545 mg sodium

SALMON AND ASPARAGUS WITH SNAP PEA SALAD

ACTIVE **10 MIN**.
TOTAL **25 MIN**.
SERVES **2**

½   bunch asparagus, trimmed on bias into 6-in. spears

2   Tbsp olive oil, divided, plus more for brushing
     Kosher salt and pepper

2   6-oz skinless salmon filets, each ¾ in. to 1 in. thick

1½   Tbsp Dijon mustard

3   Tbsp sliced chives, divided

3   oz sugar snap peas, thinly sliced on bias

2½   Tbsp roasted salted pistachios, roughly chopped

1   Tbsp tarragon leaves, chopped

½   tsp lemon zest plus 1½ Tbsp lemon juice

DIRECTIONS

1. Heat oven to 400°F. Fold four 13- by 16-in. sheets of parchment in half crosswise and unfold. Divide asparagus spears among sheets, piling on half of each sheet alongside crease. Drizzle piles with ½ Tbsp oil and season with a pinch each tsp salt and pepper.

2. Spread bottoms of salmon with half of mustard and place on top of asparagus. Spread tops with remaining mustard and sprinkle with a pinch of salt. Scatter tops with 1½ Tbsp chives. Brush empty half of parchment with oil and fold parchment over fish. Fold according to directions in sidebar.

3. Bake on rimmed baking sheet, 10 to 11 min. for medium and 13 to 14 min. for well-done.

4. Meanwhile, in a medium bowl, toss snap peas with pistachios, tarragon, lemon zest and juice, ¼ tsp salt and ⅛ tsp pepper, remaining 1½ Tbsp chives, and remaining 1½ Tbsp olive oil.

5. Open parchment packages, being very careful to avoid steam. Spoon snap pea salad on top of and around fish.

NO-FUSS FOLDING AND OPENING

TO FOLD

1. Place ingredients on half of a parchment sheet, ½ in. away from center. Fold other half over ingredients.

2. Starting at 1 end of folded side, make small overlapping folds to create half-moon shape and completely seal open sides; fold final corner underneath.

TO OPEN

Carefully tease out the folded corner, keeping your hands out of steam's way. Or, snip a cross in the center with kitchen shears and carefully pull open the cut ends.

NUTRITION

PER SERVING 480 cal, 42 g pro, 10 g carb, 4 g fiber, 4 g sugars (0 g added sugars), 30.5 g fat (5 g sat fat), 77 mg chol, 750 mg sodium

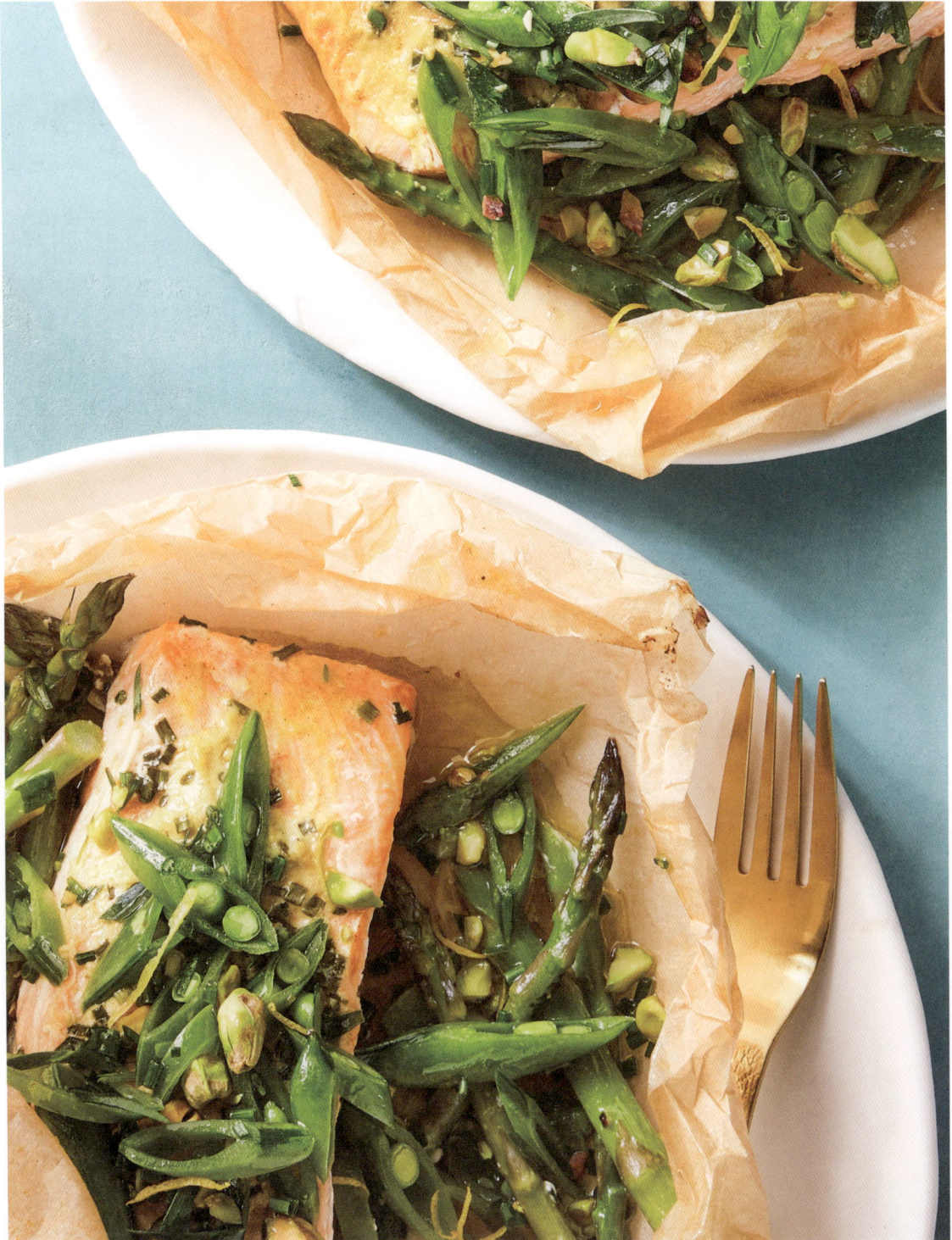

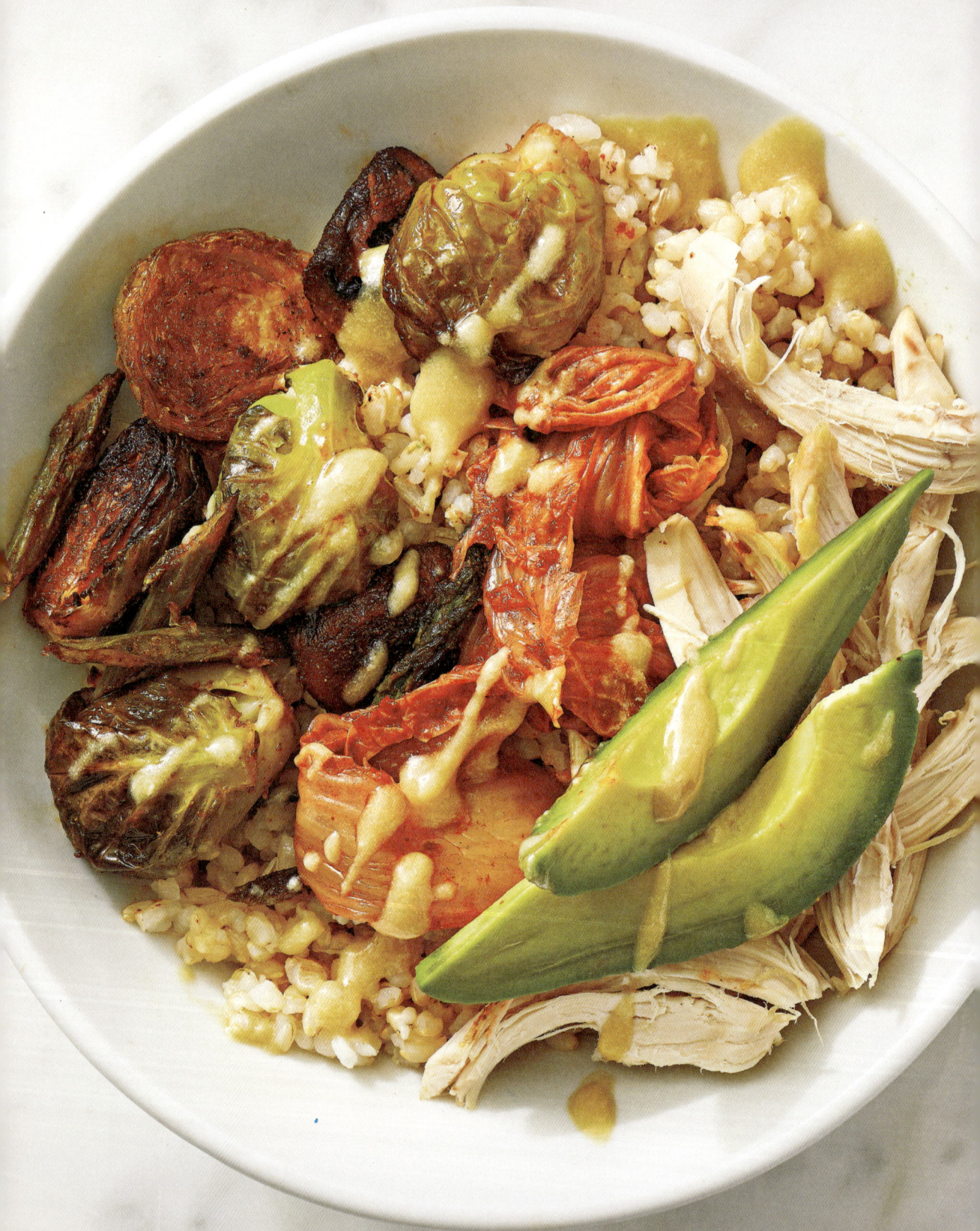

GREEN ENVY RICE BOWL

ACTIVE **10 MIN.**
TOTAL **45 MIN.**
SERVES **2**

½   lb asparagus, trimmed and chopped

½   onion, chopped

¼   lb Brussels sprouts, trimmed and halved

¼   lb cremini or button mushrooms, halved
    (quartered if large)

1   Tbsp olive oil

½   tsp ground cumin

½   tsp smoked paprika

½   tsp garlic powder
    Kosher salt

1   cup cooked brown rice

1   cup diced or shredded leftover cooked or rotisserie
    chicken (light and/or dark meat)

½   cup kimchi, optional

½   avocado, sliced

TAHINI GARLIC DRESSING

⅛   cup tahini

⅛   cup olive oil

⅛   cup apple cider vinegar

1   or 2 cloves garlic, grated

½   tsp miso paste
    Kosher salt and pepper
    Water, as necessary

DIRECTIONS

1. Heat oven to 425°F.

2. On a baking sheet, combine asparagus, onion, Brussels sprouts, and mushrooms with the olive oil, cumin, smoked paprika, garlic powder, and ½ tsp of salt. Toss once, then roast until the veggies are slightly charred, 25 to 30 min.

3. For the dressing: In a glass jar, combine the tahini, olive oil, and apple cider vinegar. Add the garlic, miso, and ⅛ tsp each salt and pepper. Thin with water to desired consistency.

4. Divide the rice among 2 bowls. Top each with half of the roasted vegetables, ½ cup chicken, ¼ cup kimchi (if using), and ¼ avocado. Drizzle with 1 Tbsp dressing each.

NUTRITION

PER SERVING 480 cal, 29 g pro, 42 g carb, 10 g fiber, 5 g sugars (0 g added sugars), 25 g fat (4 g sat fat), 60 mg chol, 930 mg sodium

CURRIED WHITE BEAN DIP

ACTIVE **10 MIN.**
TOTAL **10 MIN.**
SERVES **4 TO 6**

2   Tbsp olive oil, plus more for serving
1   large clove garlic, pressed
2   tsp curry powder
1   lemon
1   tsp lemon zest
1   15-oz can white beans, rinsed
     Kosher salt and pepper
     Cilantro, toasted pita, cucumbers, and peppers,
     for serving

DIRECTIONS

1. In a small skillet, heat oil, garlic, curry powder, and grated lemon zest until garlic is fragrant, about 2 min.

2. Transfer to a mini food processor along with white beans, 1½ Tbsp lemon juice, ¼ tsp each salt and pepper, and puree until smooth.

3. Transfer to a bowl, drizzle with additional oil, and sprinkle with cilantro. Serve with toasted pita, cucumbers, and peppers for dipping.

NUTRITION
PER SERVING 120 cal, 5 g pro, 14 g carb, 3 g fiber, 0 g sugars (0 g added sugars), 5 g fat (1 g sat fat), 0 mg chol, 260 mg sodium

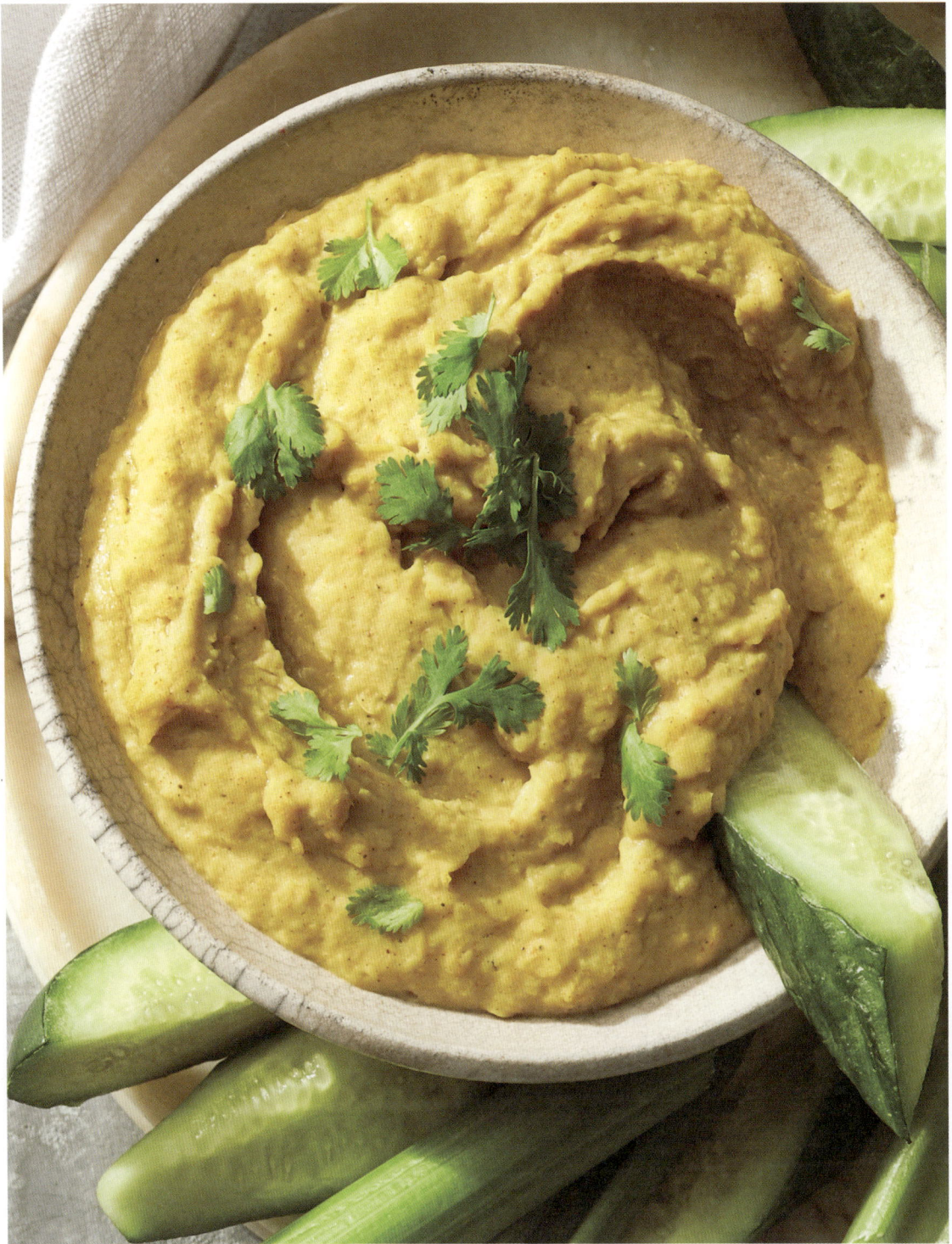

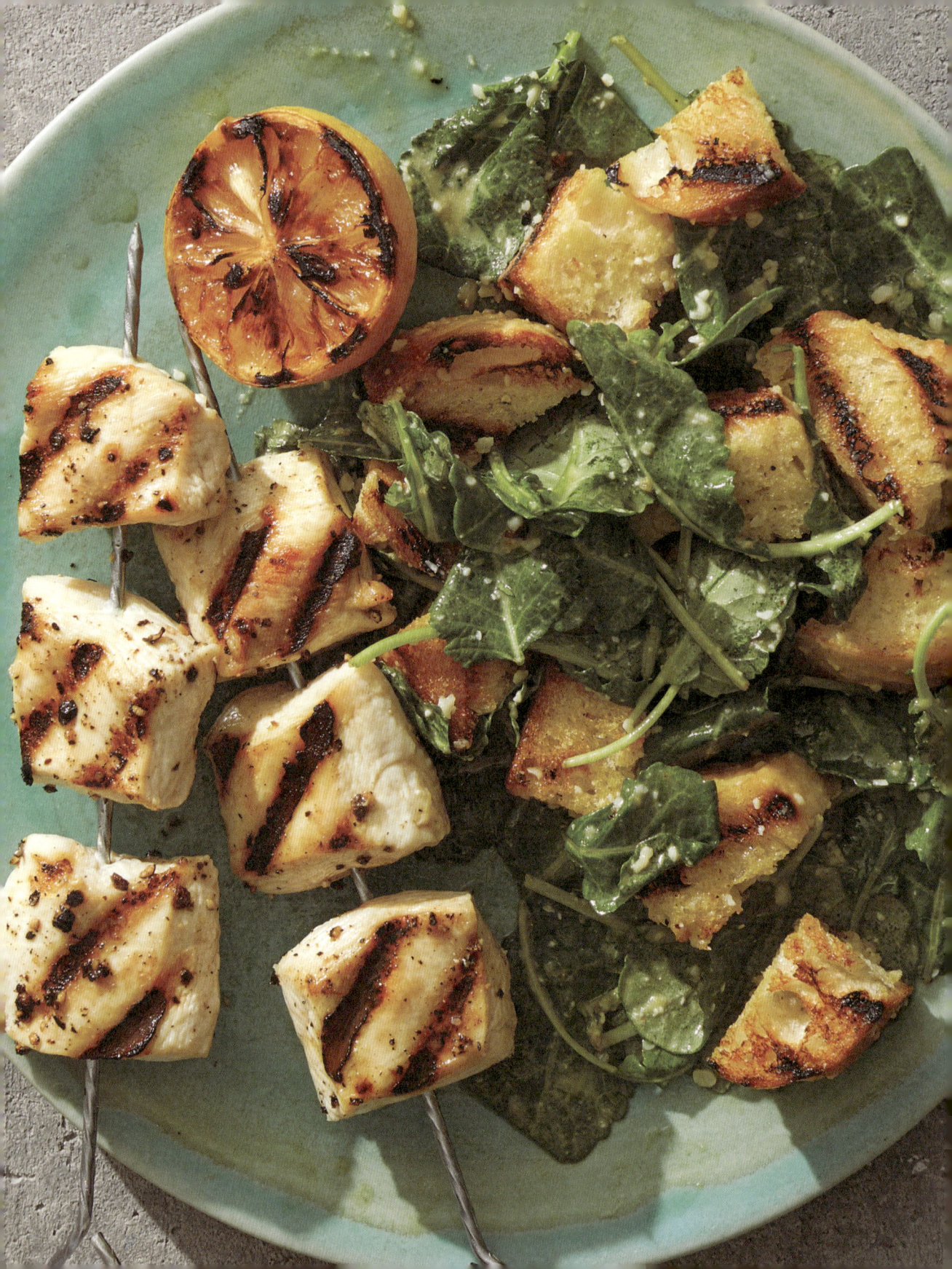

GRILLED CHICKEN SKEWERS AND KALE CAESAR

ACTIVE **25 MIN.**
TOTAL **25 MIN.**
SERVES **2**

1	lemon, halved
¾	lb boneless, skinless chicken breasts
	Kosher salt and pepper
4	thick slices baguette
½	clove garlic, halved, plus ¼ small clove garlic, finely grated
1	tsp egg yolk (from a fresh egg)
¼	tsp Dijon mustard
2½	Tbsp olive oil
⅛	cup grated Parmesan
3	cups baby kale

DIRECTIONS

1. Cut one half of the lemon in half. From remaining half, finely grate ½ tsp zest and squeeze 2 Tbsp juice, set aside.

2. Cut chicken into 1½-in. chunks; thread onto skewers and season with ⅛ tsp each salt and pepper. Grill until cooked through, 3 to 4 min. per side. Grill a quarter lemon, cut side down, until charred; squeeze over chicken. Grill bread until toasted, rub both sides with garlic halves, then cut into cubes.

3. In a large bowl, whisk together lemon zest and juice, egg yolk, mustard, grated garlic, and ¼ tsp salt. Slowly whisk in oil. Fold in Parmesan, then kale and croutons, and season with pepper. Serve with chicken.

NUTRITION
PER SERVING 490 cal, 45 g pro, 18 g carb, 1 g fiber, 2 g sugars (1 g added sugars), 26 g fat (5 g sat fat), 175 mg chol, 620 mg sodium

CURRY-AVOCADO CRISPY EGG TOAST

ACTIVE **10 MIN.**
TOTAL **10 MIN.**
SERVES **1**

¼ tsp curry powder
1½ Tbsp olive oil, divided
¼ avocado
1 tsp fresh lime juice
   Kosher salt and pepper
1 slice whole grain bread, toasted
1 large egg
1 Tbsp finely chopped cilantro

DIRECTIONS

1. In a small dry skillet on medium, toast curry powder until fragrant, 1 minute. Stir in 1 Tbsp olive oil and set aside.

2. Mash avocado with lime juice and pinch salt and spread on toast.

3. Heat remaining olive oil in a medium skillet on medium-high. Add egg and cook until whites are golden brown, crisp around the edges, and set around the yolk, about 2 min. (if edges are dark but whites are not set, remove skillet from heat; cover until whites are cooked, about 10 seconds). Season with pinch each salt and pepper.

4. Top with avocado toast with egg and chopped cilantro, then drizzle with curry oil.

NUTRITION
PER SERVING 455 cal, 13 g pro, 24 g carb, 8 g fiber, 3.5 g sugars (0 g added sugars), 34.5 g fat (6 g sat fat), 185 mg chol, 380 mg sodium

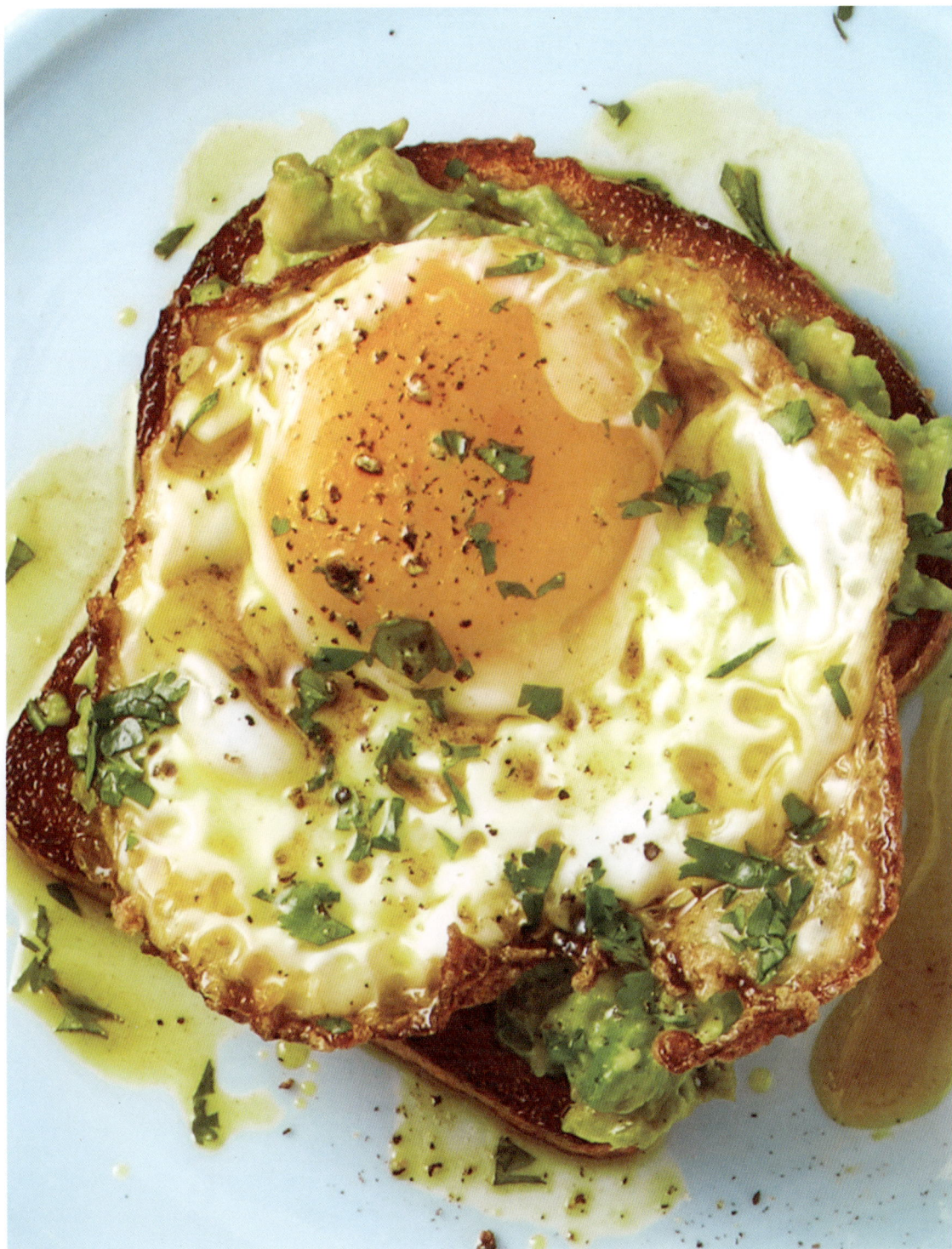

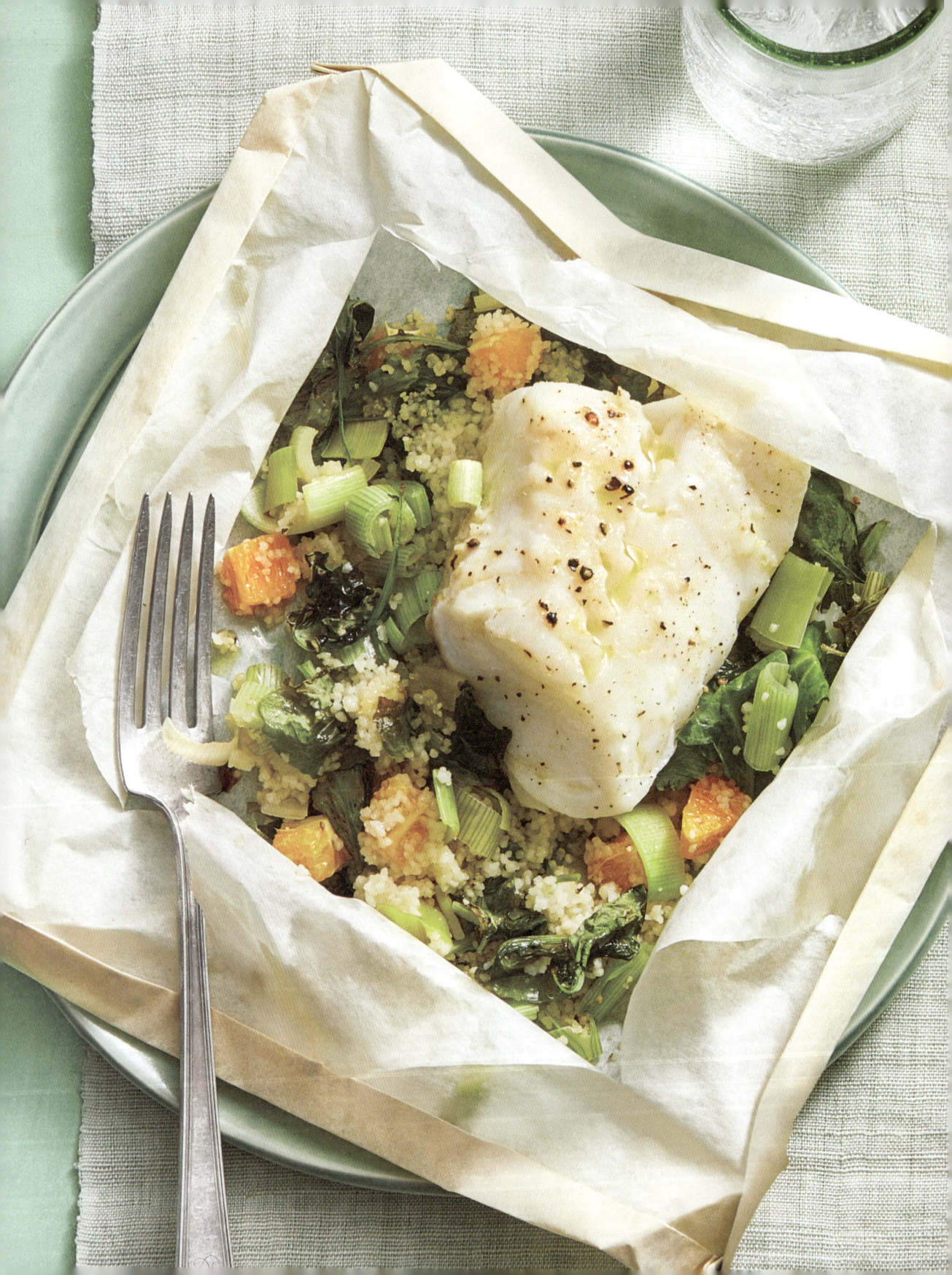

COD WITH ORANGE LEEK COUSCOUS

ACTIVE **15 MIN.**
TOTAL **30 MIN.**
SERVES **2**

½   **cup couscous**

½   **orange**

½   **leek, white and light green parts only, cut in half lengthwise, then sliced ½-in. thick**

1½   **cups baby kale**

2   **5-oz cod fillets**

½   **Tbsp olive oil**

   Kosher salt and pepper

DIRECTIONS

1. Heat oven to 425°F. Tear off eight 12-in. squares of parchment paper and arrange 4 squares on 2 baking sheets. In a medium bowl, combine couscous with ¾ cup water.

2. Cut orange in half, then peel 1 half and coarsely chop fruit. Fold orange into couscous along with leek and kale.

3. Divide couscous mixture among pieces of parchment and top each with 1 piece of cod. Drizzle with oil and sprinkle with ½ tsp salt and ¼ tsp pepper, then squeeze juice from remaining orange half over top.

4. Cover each with another piece of parchment and fold each edge up and under 3 times, tucking corner underneath (see p. 146). Roast 12 min.

5. Transfer each packet to plate. Using scissors or knife, cut an "X" in center and fold back triangles.

NUTRITION
PER SERVING 340 cal, 32 g pro, 40 g carb, 3 g fiber, 3.5 g sugars (0 g added sugars), 5 g fat (1 g sat fat), 61 mg chol, 330 mg sodium

HOMEMADE TURKEY SAUSAGE, FENNEL, AND ARUGULA WITH CHICKPEA RIGATONI

ACTIVE **25 MIN.**
TOTAL **25 MIN.**
SERVES **2**

½   lb lean ground turkey
1   tsp sweet paprika
2   cloves garlic, grated, divided
½   tsp red pepper flakes, divided
     Kosher salt and pepper
6   oz pasta (we used Banza chickpea rigatoni)
1½   Tbsp olive oil, divided
1   Tbsp fennel seeds, lightly crushed
½   large bulb fennel, cored, and thinly sliced
1   tsp fresh lemon juice
2   cups loosely packed baby arugula
2½   Tbsp grated Pecorino Romano

DIRECTIONS

1. In a bowl, combine turkey, paprika, half of garlic, ¼ tsp red pepper, and ¼ tsp salt until just fully mixed (can be made and refrigerated up to 1 day ahead).

2. Cook pasta per pkg. directions, reserving ½ cup cooking liquid before draining and rinsing

3. Meanwhile, heat 1 Tbsp oil in a large skillet on medium-high. Add fennel seeds to skillet and quickly add bits-size pieces of sausage mixture on top, gently pressing. Cook until golden brown, 5 to 6 min. Toss and cook just until cooked through, 1 to 2 min. more. Transfer to plate

4. Wipe out skillet and heat remaining ½ Tbsp oil on medium. Add sliced fennel and ⅛ tsp salt and cook, stirring occasionally, until just tender, about 4 min. Stir in lemon juice, ¼ cup reserved pasta cooking liquid, and remaining ¼ tsp red pepper.

5. Gently fold pasta and arugula into fennel mixture, then half of sausage, adding more cooking liquid if pasta seems dry. Serve topped with remaining sausage and Pecorino Romano.

NUTRITION

PER SERVING 645 cal, 47 g pro, 59 g carb, 12 g fiber, 7 g sugars (0 g added sugars), 29 g fat (6 g sat fat), 97 mg chol, 730 mg sodium

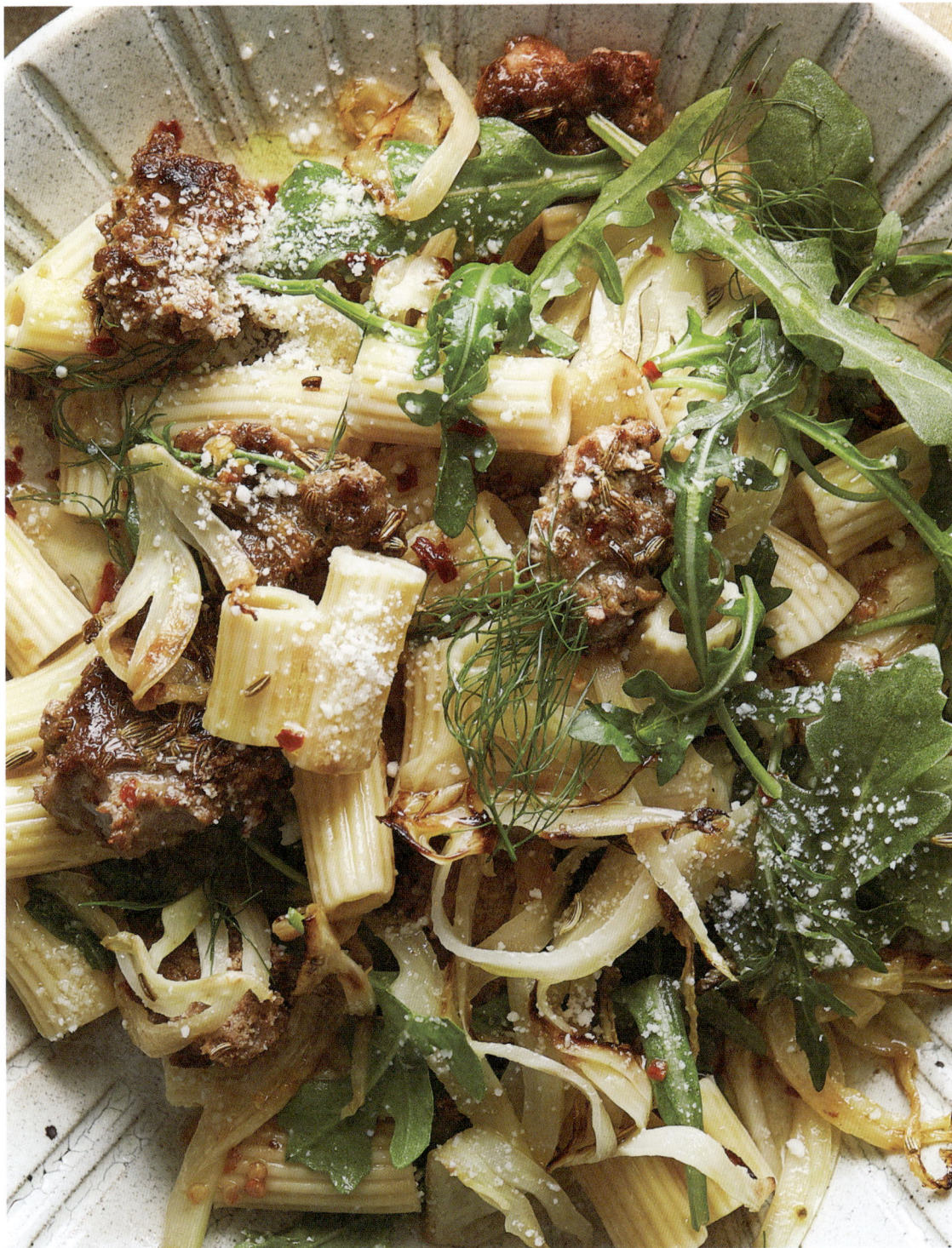

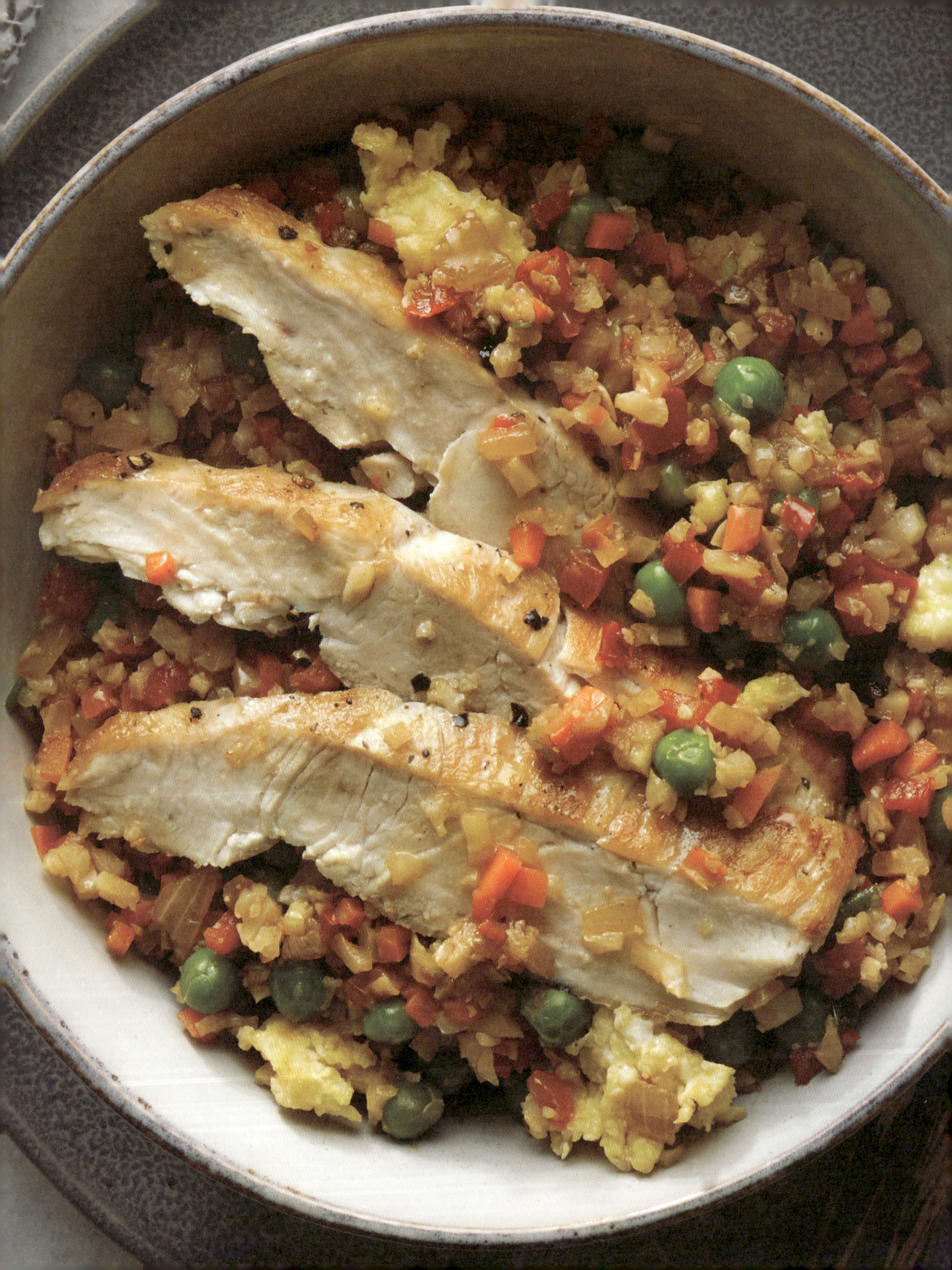

CHICKEN WITH FRIED CAULIFLOWER RICE

ACTIVE **10 MIN.**
TOTAL **35 MIN.**
SERVES **2**

½   Tbsp plus 1 tsp grapeseed oil, divided

½   lb boneless, skinless chicken breasts, pounded to even thickness

2   large eggs, beaten

1   red pepper, finely chopped

1   small carrot, finely chopped

½   small onion, finely chopped

1   clove garlic, finely chopped

2   scallions, finely chopped, plus more for serving

½   cup frozen peas, thawed

2   cups cauliflower "rice"

1   Tbsp low-sodium soy sauce

1   tsp rice vinegar

Kosher salt and pepper

DIRECTIONS

1. Heat a large, deep skillet over medium-high. Add ½ Tbsp oil, then chicken and cook until golden brown, 3 to 4 min. per side; transfer to a cutting board and let rest for 6 min. before slicing.

2. Add 1 tsp oil to skillet, then eggs, and scramble until just set, 1 to 2 min.; transfer to a bowl.

3. Add red pepper, carrot, and onion and cook, stirring often until just tender, 4 to 5 min. Stir in garlic and cook, 1 minute. Toss with scallions and peas.

4. Add cauliflower, soy sauce, and rice vinegar and toss to combine. Then let the cauliflower sit, without stirring, until beginning to brown 2 to 3 min. Toss with sliced chicken, eggs, and ⅛ tsp each salt and pepper.

NUTRITION
PER SERVING 340 cal, 34 g pro, 18 g carb, 6 g fiber, 6 g sugars (0 g added sugars), 13 g fat (2.5 g sat fat), 230 mg chol, 500 mg sodium

GREEN PINEAPPLE COCONUT SMOOTHIE

ACTIVE **10 MIN.**
TOTAL **10 MIN.**
SERVES **1**

½   cup light coconut milk
½   Tbsp lime juice
½   tsp grated lime zest
1   cup baby spinach
½   cup frozen pineapple chunks
½   banana, sliced and frozen

DIRECTIONS
In a blender, combine all ingredients and puree until smooth.

NUTRITION
PER SERVING 190 cal, 4 g pro, 30 g carb, 4 g fiber, 11.5g sugars (0 g added sugars), 7 g fat (7 g sat fat), 0 mg chol, 45 mg sodium

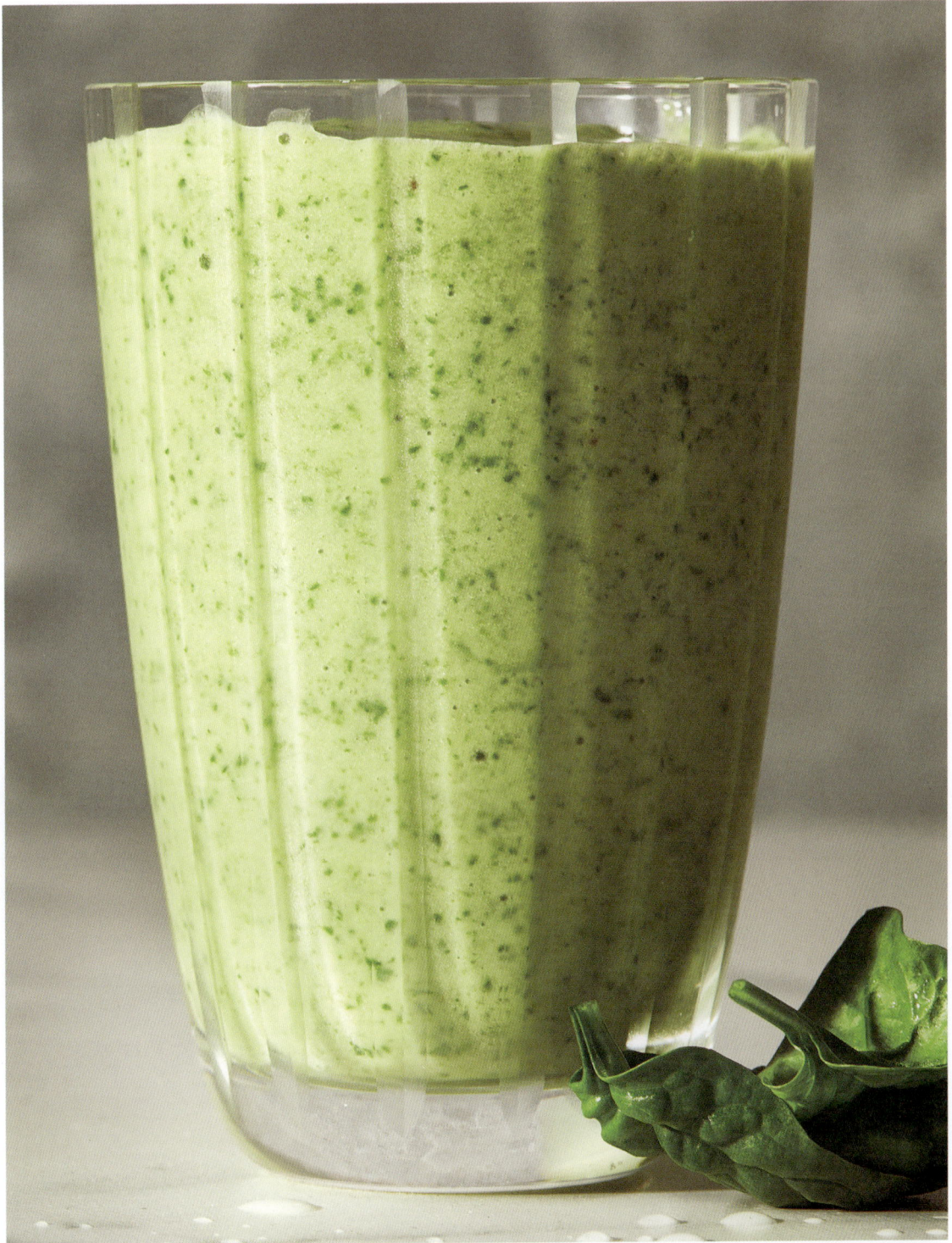

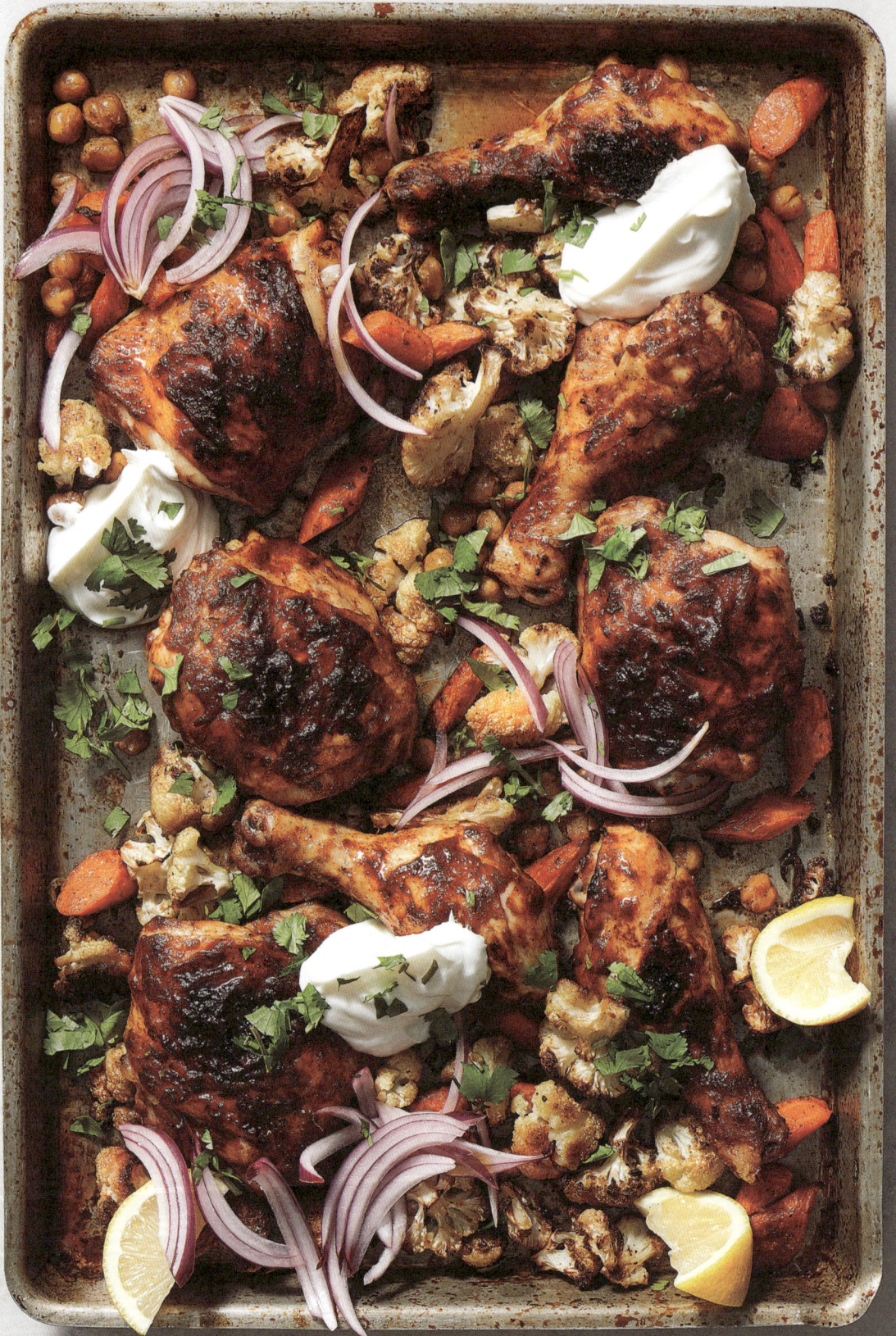

SHEET PAN CHICKEN TIKKA WITH CAULIFLOWER AND CHICKPEAS

ACTIVE **25 MIN.**
TOTAL **50 MIN.**
SERVES **2**

2	small chicken legs, split
½	cup jarred tikka masala sauce
¼	medium cauliflower, cut into small florets
6	oz carrots, cut into ¾-in. chunks
½	cup canned chickpeas, rinsed
½	Tbsp olive oil
½	tsp garam masala
	Kosher salt and pepper
¼	red onion
⅛	cup low-fat yogurt
⅛	cup cilantro, chopped
	Lemon wedges, for serving

DIRECTIONS

1. Place chicken and tikka masala sauce in a resealable plastic bag. Seal and toss to coat; let sit 30 min. or refrigerate overnight.

2. Heat oven to 425°F. On a large rimmed baking sheet, toss cauliflower, carrots, and chickpeas with oil, garam masala, and ¼ tsp each salt and pepper.

3. Remove chicken from bag, letting excess marinade drip off, and nestle among vegetables; discard marinade. Roast until chicken is cooked through, 30 to 35 min.

4. Meanwhile, thinly slice onion, transfer to a bowl, cover with water, and let soak 10 min.; drain well. Serve chicken topped with onion, yogurt, and cilantro. Serve with lemon wedges.

NUTRITION
PER SERVING 575 cal, 55 g pro, 27 g carb, 7 g fiber, 13 g sugars (0.5 g added sugars), 27.5 g fat (7 g sat fat), 110 mg chol, 810 mg sodium

MEAL PLAN
BONUS TRACKER

BREAKFAST

SNACK

LUNCH

SNACK

DINNER

WATER

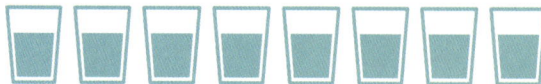

MOVEMENT Y ☐ N ☐

ACTIVITY	DURATION	INTENSITY

SLEEP

BEDTIME	WAKE UP

MOOD

☺ ☻ ☹

MEAL PLAN
BONUS TRACKER

BREAKFAST

SNACK

LUNCH

SNACK

DINNER

WATER

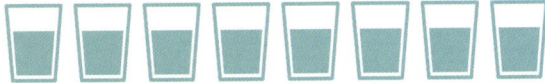

MOVEMENT Y☐ N☐

ACTIVITY	DURATION	INTENSITY

SLEEP

BEDTIME	WAKE UP

MOOD

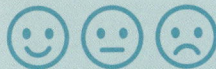

MEAL PLAN
BONUS TRACKER

BREAKFAST

SNACK

LUNCH

SNACK

DINNER

WATER

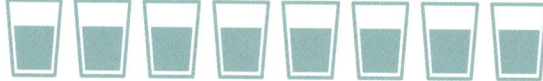

MOVEMENT Y ☐ N ☐

ACTIVITY	DURATION	INTENSITY

SLEEP

BEDTIME	WAKE UP

MOOD

☺ ☺ ☹

MEAL PLAN
BONUS TRACKER

BREAKFAST

SNACK

LUNCH

SNACK

DINNER

WATER

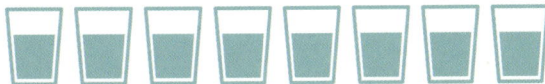

MOVEMENT Y ☐ N ☐

ACTIVITY	DURATION	INTENSITY

SLEEP

BEDTIME	WAKE UP

MOOD

☺ ☺ ☹

MEAL PLAN
BONUS TRACKER

BREAKFAST

SNACK

LUNCH

SNACK

DINNER

WATER

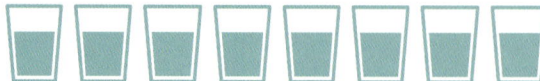

MOVEMENT Y ☐ N ☐

ACTIVITY	DURATION	INTENSITY

SLEEP

BEDTIME	WAKE UP

MOOD

☺ 😐 ☹

Credits

INTERIOR PHOTOGRAPHY

andresr/E+/Getty Images: 35; PictureNet Corporation/Getty Images: 176; Chris Court: 71; Danielle Daly: 48, 155, 167; DragonImages/Adobe Stock Images: 30; Philip Friedman: 7, 47, 97, 127, 164; FomaA/Adobe Stock Images: 106 (chicken); Mike Garten: 56, 64, 68, 85-89, 93, 98-101, 115-116, 120-124, 128-131, 135, 147-152, 156-160; Brierley Horton, M.S., R.D.: 3; Akira Ito/Adobe Stock Images: 106 (brown rice); kerkezz/Adobe Stock Images: 12; Erika Lapresto: 52-55, 63; LILECHKA75/Getty Images: 72; lukesw/Adobe Stock Images: 26; Charles Masters: 94; mizina/Adobe Stock Images: 17, 21; Paolese/Adobe Stock Images: 18; Pixel-Shot/Adobe Stock Images: 14; Con Poulos: 60; Prostock-studio/Adobe Stock Images: 25; Armando Rafael: 90, 119, 163; Nelea Reazanteva/Adobe Stock Images: 76 (pistachios); Robert/Adobe Stock Images: 10; santypan/iStock/Getty Images: 9; Lucy Schaeffer: 59, 102; Africa Studio/Adobe Stock Images: 38 (hard-boiled eggs and carrots); Christopher Testani: 67, 132, 168; Liliya Trott/Adobe Stock Images: 16; vaaseenaa/Adobe Stock Images: 6; valentinamaslova/Adobe Stock Images: 27; VICUSCHKA/Adobe Stock Images: 22; Westend61/Getty Images: 15; whyframeshot/Adobe Stock Images: 29; Carolyn Williams, Ph.D., R.D.: 3; Romulo Yanes: 51

RECIPE DEVELOPMENT

The Prevention Test Kitchen: 49-57, 61-66, 70, 84, 88-95, 99-100, 114-122, 126, 133, 146, 153-154, 158-161, 166-169; The Good Housekeeping Test Kitchen: 129; Marci Herman: 125; Heather K. Jones: 87, Kristina Kurek: 58, 103, 149, 162; Tina Martinez: 69, 134; Kate Merker: 69, 130, 134, 157; Sarah Mirkin, R.D.N.: 46, 73, 96, 165; Taylor Murray: 157

This book is intended as a reference volume only, not as a medical manual. The information given here is designed to help you make informed decisions about your health. It is not intended as a substitute for any treatment that may have been prescribed by your doctor. If you suspect that you have a medical problem, we urge you to seek competent medical help.

Mention of specific companies, organizations, or authorities in this book does not imply endorsement by the author or publisher, nor does mention of specific companies, organizations, or authorities imply that they endorse this book, its author, or the publisher.

Internet addresses and telephone numbers given in this book were accurate at the time it went to press.

Cover photography by Mike Garten
Book design by Caroline Pickering

Library of Congress Cataloging-in-Publication Data is on file with the publisher.

ISBN 978-1-955710-28-2

Printed in China

2 4 6 8 10 9 7 5 3 1 paperback

HEARST

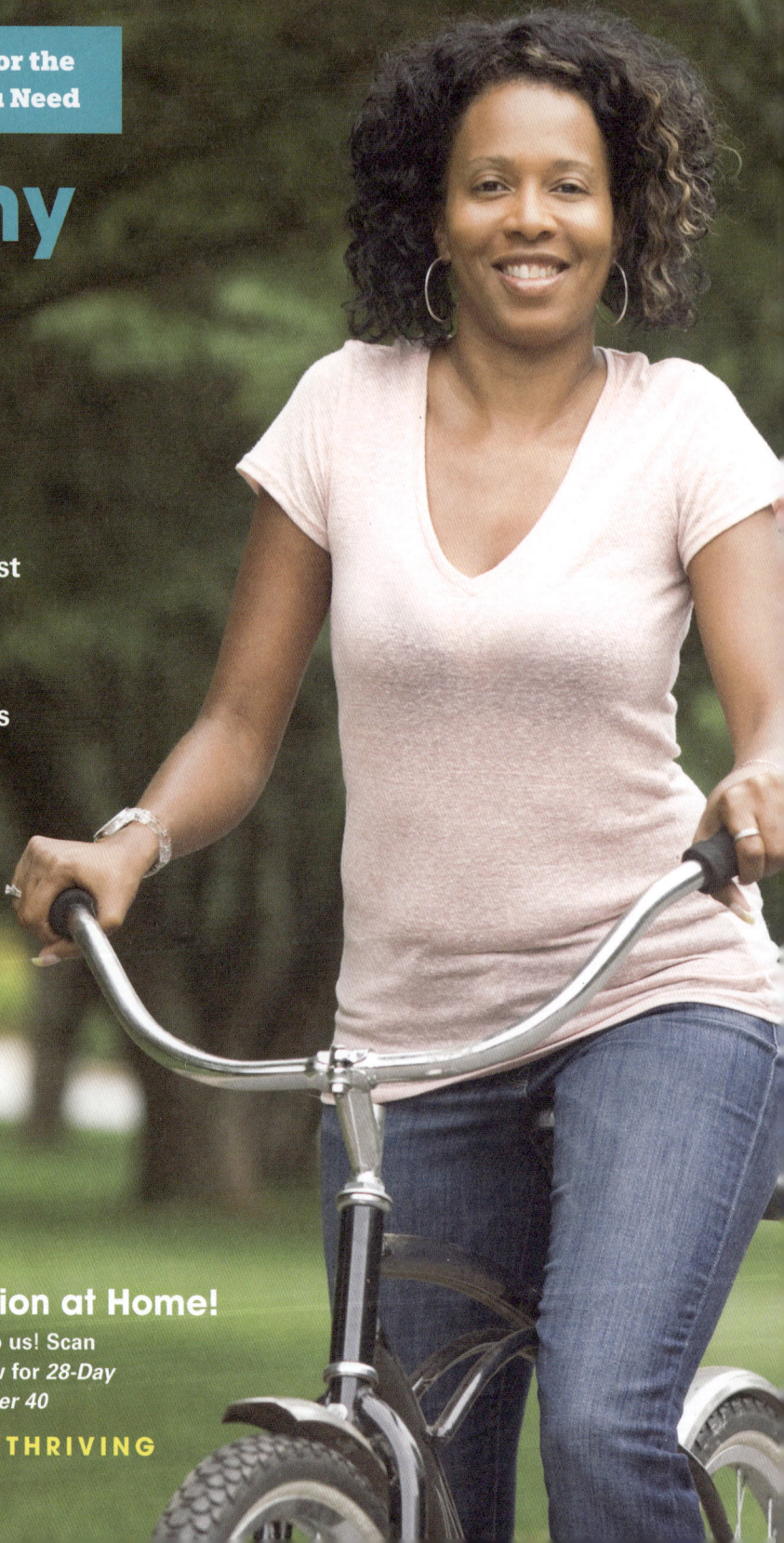